BEYOND BOUNDARIES: 101 Practical Tips for Special Needs Parenting

Brenda Maye

TABLE OF CONTENTS

INTRODUCTION

Welcome, weary yet determined traveler, to a journey that will take you beyond the known horizons of parenting. This book, "Beyond Boundaries: 101 Practical Tips for Special Needs Parenting," is not your typical guide. It is a compass, a lifeline, and a lantern to illuminate the path that stretches before you as you embark on the extraordinary adventure of raising a child with special needs.

I am your fellow voyager, a fellow parent who has traversed the twisting trails, the unexpected turns, and the soaring heights that this unique journey offers. Just like you, I've navigated the vast terrain of emotions – from the depths of uncertainty to the peaks of profound joy and love. And through it all, I've discovered that embracing this extraordinary expedition requires courage, resilience, and an open heart.

When my own journey began, I found myself standing at a crossroads, perplexed and overwhelmed. The diagnosis came like a tempest, leaving me drenched in fear and uncertainty. But as the storm subsided, I realized that this was not the end; it was a new beginning. My child's special needs became the coordinates for an uncharted voyage, and as I set sail, I discovered that there were no boundaries to our love, our dreams, or our possibilities.

In these pages, you will find a treasure trove of practical tips, garnered not only from my own experiences but from a vast community of parents, professionals, and advocates who have dedicated themselves to illuminating the path for others like us. These insights are not just generic platitudes but tried-and-tested strategies that have weathered the toughest of storms.

Every parent knows that there's no handbook for raising a child – no magic spell or secret formula that guarantees smooth sailing. But as parents of extraordinary children, we have an opportunity to redefine what it means to embrace the unknown with open arms. We become pioneers, forging a path through the uncharted territory of love, compassion, and understanding.

Throughout this book, we'll delve into the early years of diagnosis and intervention, seeking out a support network that becomes a lifeline in the darkest of times. We'll explore how to create an inclusive home environment that fosters growth, development, and joy. We'll navigate the intricate waters of education, advocating for individualized plans that nurture our children's potential. We'll address the unique challenges of health and wellness, diving into the world of sensory integration, and discovering the magic of play.

And as we journey further, we'll set our sights on the horizon of adulthood, preparing for the transition that awaits our children when they spread their wings and soar toward independence. We'll explore the legal and financial aspects of special needs parenting, arming ourselves with the knowledge to secure the brightest possible future for our beloved children.

Yet, this is more than just a book about parenting. It is a celebration of the human spirit, the boundless resilience that dwells within each of us, and the unyielding strength that emerges from the depths of our hearts. As we embrace our child's special needs, we uncover the superpowers that lie dormant within them and ourselves.

Dear reader, I hope this book becomes a beacon of hope and a guiding light for you, illuminating your path when the night seems darkest. My wish is that you discover not only practical tips but also the inspiration to embrace every challenge and triumph as you journey beyond boundaries.

So, let us hoist our sails and set forth on this transformative adventure together. As we traverse uncharted waters, let us remember that there is no map to guide us, but we have something far more potent – love, strength, and a community of fellow adventurers to share in the triumphs and tribulations. Together, let us journey beyond boundaries and discover the extraordinary beauty that lies on the other side.

Bon voyage, dear parent, bon voyage.

CHAPTER 1

Understanding Special Needs Parenting

1.1 What Are Special Needs?

When we speak of special needs parenting, we embark on a journey that transcends the boundaries of conventional parenting. It is a path that leads us to explore uncharted territories, navigating through a landscape of challenges and joys unique to each child and family. At its essence, special needs parenting involves caring for and nurturing children who require extra support due to physical, developmental, emotional, or cognitive differences.

Special needs encompass a broad spectrum of conditions, and each child's journey is as individual as the stars in the night sky. These needs may arise from various factors, including genetic conditions, birth injuries, neurological disorders, sensory processing issues, learning disabilities, and chronic health conditions. Some children may have multiple needs, making their journeys even more intricate and extraordinary.

As parents of children with special needs, we must first embrace the truth that every child is an exceptional being, gifted with their own set of abilities and challenges. These challenges should never define them but rather become the fuel that ignites their unique light, illuminating the world in ways we could never have imagined.

1.2 Embracing the Journey

The moment we discover that our child has special needs, our world undergoes a seismic shift. Emotions surge like waves in a tumultuous sea—fear, confusion, sadness, and even relief, as we finally have a name for the difficulties our child faces. It is a moment that etches itself into our hearts forever.

As we stand at the crossroads of this new reality, we may find ourselves grappling with a plethora of questions. Will we be able to provide the support our child needs? How will our family dynamics change? What kind of future awaits our beloved child? These questions are not meant to be answered all at once, for this journey is not a sprint; it is a marathon of love, courage, and resilience.

Embracing the special needs parenting journey requires us to shed preconceived notions of what parenting should be. It beckons us to step outside our comfort zones and let go of any sense of control we once believed we had. Instead, we learn to dance in sync with the rhythm of our child's unique song, understanding that the melody may change, but the love remains constant.

In this journey, we are not alone. We are accompanied by an extraordinary community of parents, caregivers, therapists, educators, and advocates who have walked similar paths before us. These fellow travelers become our allies, our guides, and our lifelines when the path seems insurmountable. Together, we form a bond forged by shared experiences, understanding nods, and the unwavering belief that our children can and will thrive.

It is essential to remember that this journey is not without its moments of beauty and triumph. In celebrating our child's successes, no matter how small, we learn the true meaning of joy. We witness the resilience of the human spirit, the strength of our child's determination, and the magic that unfolds when we embrace each milestone with open arms.

1.3 Advocating for Your Child

As parents of children with special needs, we often find ourselves wearing the mantle of advocate. We become champions for our child's rights, needs, and potential, navigating complex systems, and breaking barriers that hinder their progress. Advocacy becomes an art we must master, a powerful tool in ensuring that our children receive the support and opportunities they deserve.

One of the first and most crucial steps in advocacy is educating ourselves about our child's specific needs and conditions. This knowledge empowers us to make informed decisions, communicate effectively with professionals, and actively participate in crafting an individualized plan to support our child's growth and development.

Communication becomes the cornerstone of effective advocacy. We learn to articulate our child's strengths, challenges and needs to educators, healthcare providers, and other members of the support team. Sharing our insights and observations is essential in creating a holistic understanding of our child, paving the way for collaborative solutions.

However, advocacy goes beyond speaking for our children; it also involves listening. By actively listening to our child's desires, interests, and preferences, we can better tailor the support and interventions they receive. Our child becomes an equal partner in this journey, their voice amplifying the chorus of advocacy that surrounds them.

In some instances, advocating for our child may require us to challenge established norms or systems. We may need to break down barriers to access quality education, inclusive environments, and medical care. This is not always an easy path, and it may be fraught with obstacles, but the fire of determination within us fuels our unwavering commitment to securing the best opportunities for our child.

As advocates, we find strength in unity. Connecting with local and online support groups, parent networks, and advocacy organizations empowers us with valuable resources, knowledge, and a network of like-minded individuals. These communities provide a safe space to share experiences, seek advice, and celebrate victories, creating a powerful force for change.

Throughout this journey, self-advocacy is equally important. As parents, we may face burnout, feelings of isolation, and a range of emotions that require attention. Taking care of our well-being enables us to be the best advocates for our children, so self-compassion and seeking support when needed are vital parts of the journey.

In conclusion, special needs parenting is a transformative voyage that stretches the boundaries of our hearts and minds. It is a journey where we celebrate the unique light our children bring to the world and embrace the challenges as opportunities for growth and learning. Advocacy becomes our compass, guiding us through uncharted waters, ensuring that our children's voices are heard, and their dreams become reality. Together, we discover that the power of love, understanding, and advocacy knows no bounds, and it empowers us to create a world where every child can shine bright, regardless of their unique needs.

CHAPTER 2

Diagnosis and Early Intervention

The journey of special needs parenting often begins with the critical phase of diagnosis and early intervention. This chapter delves into the process of identifying developmental delays, seeking professional help, and creating an early intervention plan. These initial steps are the foundation upon which we build a framework of support and understanding for our children, setting them on a path toward reaching their full potential.

2.1 Identifying Developmental Delays

In the vast spectrum of child development, each milestone achieved is a moment of celebration for parents. From the first smile to those tentative steps, we eagerly watch our children grow and thrive. However, when our child's development deviates from the typical trajectory, we may begin to notice signs of developmental delays. Identifying these delays early is essential, as it allows for timely intervention, which can significantly impact a child's progress and future outcomes.

Developmental delays can manifest in various areas, including:

1. Cognitive Development: Difficulty with problem-solving, learning, memory, and understanding concepts appropriate for their age.

2. Gross Motor Skills: Delays in achieving physical milestones such as crawling, walking, or jumping.

3. Fine Motor Skills: Challenges with tasks that require hand-eye coordination, such as holding a pencil, tying shoelaces, or buttoning a shirt.

4. Speech and Language: Difficulty in expressing themselves verbally, understanding spoken language, or forming sentences.

5. Social and Emotional Development: Struggles in social interactions, forming relationships, or understanding and expressing emotions.

6. Adaptive Skills: Challenges in performing daily activities independently, such as dressing, eating, and personal hygiene.

Recognizing developmental delays can be an emotionally challenging experience for parents. It is essential to remember that seeking professional evaluation is not a reflection of failure or inadequacy as a parent. Rather, it is an act of love and dedication to ensuring our child receives the support they need to flourish.

Observing and documenting our child's behavior and developmental milestones is an invaluable step in the identification process. Keeping a journal of observations and discussing concerns with other caregivers or family members can provide valuable insights. Additionally, familiarizing ourselves with typical developmental milestones for our child's age and engaging in activities that support their growth can help in recognizing delays.

Every child is unique, and developmental milestones can vary widely, but there are general guidelines provided by healthcare professionals and child development experts. If we notice significant deviations from these milestones or have persistent concerns, seeking a professional evaluation is the next crucial step.

2.2 Seeking Professional Help

When we suspect developmental delays in our child, it is essential to connect with qualified professionals who specialize in child development and related fields. The journey toward a diagnosis may involve multiple assessments and evaluations, but these steps are vital in gaining a comprehensive understanding of our child's strengths, challenges, and needs.

The first point of contact is often our child's pediatrician or primary healthcare provider. They can conduct an initial assessment and may refer us to specialists such as pediatric developmental specialists, pediatric neurologists, psychologists, speech-language pathologists, occupational therapists, or physical therapists.

The evaluation process may include:

1. Developmental Screenings: These are brief assessments designed to identify potential developmental delays in areas such as communication, gross motor skills, fine motor skills, and social interactions.

2. Comprehensive Assessments: These evaluations involve in-depth assessments conducted by specialists to gather a more comprehensive picture of our child's strengths and areas of concern. These assessments may involve standardized tests, observations, and parent interviews.

3. Medical Evaluations: Some developmental delays may be related to medical conditions or genetic disorders. In such cases, medical evaluations by pediatric specialists are essential for accurate diagnosis and appropriate medical management.

4. Psychological Assessments: Psychological evaluations can provide valuable insights into cognitive functioning, emotional well-being, and behavioral patterns.

As parents, it is essential to actively participate in the evaluation process, sharing our observations, concerns, and insights with the professionals involved. We are the experts on our child's behaviors, personality, and experiences, and our input is invaluable in formulating a holistic understanding of our child.

The process of seeking professional help and undergoing evaluations can be emotionally taxing, but it is a pivotal step in providing the best possible support for our child. The diagnosis, when it comes, does not define our child but rather opens doors to specialized interventions and opportunities for growth.

Once we have received a diagnosis or a clearer understanding of our child's developmental needs, we enter the realm of early intervention.

2.3 Creating an Early Intervention Plan

Early intervention is a cornerstone of support for children with developmental delays. It refers to a range of targeted services and therapies designed to address the unique needs of young children and set them on a trajectory of positive growth and development. The concept of "early" intervention is based on the understanding that the developing brain is highly malleable during the early years, making it a critical window for maximizing the benefits of intervention.

Creating an early intervention plan involves a collaborative effort between parents, healthcare professionals, therapists, educators, and other support providers. This personalized plan aims to address the specific developmental areas where our child requires assistance and support.

The components of an early intervention plan may include:

1. **Individualized Goals**: Based on the assessment findings, the intervention team works with parents to set specific, measurable, achievable, relevant, and time-bound (SMART) goals for the child. These goals are tailored to address their unique strengths and areas of need.

2. **Targeted Therapies**: Early intervention may involve various therapies, depending on the child's needs. Some common therapies include:
   - a. Speech-Language Therapy: Addresses speech and language delays, communication challenges, and articulation difficulties.
   - b. Occupational Therapy: Focuses on fine motor skills, sensory processing, and activities of daily living.
   - c. Physical Therapy: Aims to improve gross motor skills, mobility, and coordination.
   - d. Behavioral Therapy: Addresses behavioral challenges, social skills, and emotional regulation.
   - e. Play Therapy: Utilizes play as a means of communication and emotional expression.

3. **Parent Education and Training**: As primary caregivers, parents play a pivotal role in their child's development. Early intervention programs often provide parent education and training sessions, equipping parents with strategies and techniques to support their child's progress at home.

4. **Inclusive Early Education**: Early intervention often includes participation in inclusive early education settings. These environments provide opportunities for children with developmental delays to interact with typically developing peers, fostering socialization and learning.

5. **Transition Planning**: As the child approaches preschool age, transition planning becomes crucial. This involves preparing the child and family for the transition from early intervention services to preschool programs.

6. **Family-Centered Approach**: Successful early intervention embraces a family-centered approach, recognizing that families are a child's primary source of support and care. The intervention team works collaboratively with the family, respecting their values, priorities, and cultural background.

7. **Ongoing Monitoring and Assessment**: Early intervention is not a one-time event but rather an ongoing process. Regular monitoring and assessments help track the child's progress, make necessary adjustments to the intervention plan, and celebrate milestones achieved.

Early intervention is not a linear path, and progress may vary for each child. It requires patience, perseverance, and open communication with the intervention team. As parents, we play a vital role in advocating for our child's needs and ensuring that the early intervention plan is dynamic, responsive, and inclusive.

In conclusion, the journey of diagnosis and early intervention is a profound and transformative experience for parents of children with developmental delays. It is a journey that requires courage, resilience, and a willingness to embrace the uniqueness of our children.

Identifying developmental delays early empowers us to seek professional help and create an early intervention plan that becomes a roadmap to our child's success and happiness. As we embark on this journey hand-in-hand with our children, we recognize that every step we take is a step toward unlocking their incredible potential and nurturing their brightest future.

CHAPTER 3

Building a Support Network

Parenting is a remarkable and rewarding journey, but it can also be challenging and overwhelming at times. When we have children with special needs, the journey takes on new dimensions, and the need for support becomes even more critical.

Building a robust support network is like creating a safety net that catches us when we stumble, lifts us when we fail, and celebrates with us when we succeed. In this chapter, we explore the invaluable role of support groups, the camaraderie of connecting with other parents, and the strength that comes from involving family and friends in the journey of special needs parenting.

3.1 Engaging with Support Groups

In the labyrinth of special needs parenting, finding others who share our journey can be a beacon of hope and understanding. Support groups are like oases amidst the vast desert, where we can find solace, empathy, and the collective wisdom of parents who have navigated similar challenges. Engaging with support groups is a powerful means of connecting with like-minded individuals who can relate to our experiences and offer invaluable insights and encouragement.

Support groups for parents of children with special needs come in various forms, such as in-person meetings, online forums, social media groups, and community organizations. These groups may be specific to a particular condition, disability, or age group, while others may be more general, encompassing a diverse range of special needs.

The benefits of engaging with support groups are manifold:

1. **Shared Experiences**: Support groups provide a safe space for parents to share their journeys, challenges, triumphs, and emotions without fear of judgment. Here, we find others who understand the unique experiences and complexities of special needs parenting.

2. **Information and Resources**: Support groups serve as valuable repositories of knowledge, resources, and information about various therapies, interventions, educational options, and community services. Parents can exchange ideas and learn from each other's experiences.

3. **Emotional Support**: Parenting a child with special needs can be emotionally taxing. In support groups, we find a network of empathetic listeners who can offer

comfort, encouragement, and a shoulder to lean on during difficult times.

4. **Advocacy**: Collective advocacy becomes more potent when parents join forces through support groups. Together, we can advocate for better policies, services, and inclusivity for our children and the special needs community as a whole.

5. **Reducing Isolation**: Special needs parenting can be isolating, as it may be challenging for others to fully grasp the nuances of our journey. Support groups provide a sense of belonging and camaraderie, reducing feelings of isolation.

6. **Celebrating Milestones**: In support groups, every milestone, no matter how small, becomes a shared victory. Celebrating achievements, big or small, creates a sense of celebration and encouragement.

When engaging with support groups, it is essential to find a community that aligns with our values, beliefs, and needs. Some groups may be more focused on problem-solving and providing practical advice, while others may emphasize emotional support and sharing personal experiences. The ideal support group will strike a balance that resonates with each individual's preferences and requirements.

3.2 Connecting with Other Parents

A shared experience is a bond that connects people in the most profound ways. Connecting with other parents who are on similar journeys as ours creates a unique and meaningful sense of community. These connections often happen organically, be it at school, therapy sessions, community events, or support group meetings. Developing friendships with other parents opens the door to a world of mutual support and understanding.

The benefits of connecting with other parents are profound:

1. **Empathy and Understanding**: Other parents who have walked a similar path can empathize with our challenges and understand the rollercoaster of emotions that accompany special needs parenting.

2. **Exchange of Ideas**: Sharing experiences and perspectives with other parents can lead to a rich exchange of ideas, strategies, and approaches to parenting and supporting our children.

3. **Playdates and Socialization**: Facilitating playdates and social interactions with other children who have special needs can create an inclusive environment where children can relate to each other's experiences.

4. **Problem-Solving**: When we encounter specific challenges, discussing them with other parents may lead to creative problem-solving and new insights.

5. **Collaboration and Advocacy**: Joining forces with other parents allows us to become a unified and powerful voice in advocating for the needs of our children and the special needs community.

While connecting with other parents can be an incredibly positive experience, it is essential to remember that each family's journey is unique. Parents may have different beliefs, approaches, and experiences, and it is crucial to respect and honor these differences while appreciating the shared bond of special needs parenting.

Online platforms and social media have become valuable tools for connecting with other parents, regardless of geographical distance. Social media groups and forums provide a virtual space where parents can share stories, ask questions, and find support from parents across the globe. However, it is essential to approach online interactions with discernment, as the information shared may not always be accurate or applicable to individual situations.

Creating and nurturing friendships with other parents may require some effort and stepping out of one's comfort zone, but the rewards are immeasurable. These connections serve as a lifeline, fostering a sense of belonging and support that weaves a safety net for our families.

3.3 Involving Family and Friends

Family and friends form the bedrock of our support system. They are our pillars of strength, love, and unwavering belief in our children's potential. Involving family and friends in the journey of special needs parenting is not only beneficial for us as parents but also creates a network of care and understanding for our children.

Here are ways to involve family and friends in the journey:

1. **Open Communication**: Transparent and open communication is the foundation of involving family and friends. Share information about your child's condition, strengths, challenges, and needs. Educate them about the nature of special needs, so they have a deeper understanding.

2. **Awareness and Sensitivity**: Encourage family members and friends to become aware of and sensitive to the unique needs and preferences of your child. Understanding the impact of sensory issues, communication challenges, or behavioral differences can foster a supportive environment.

3. **Hands-On Support**: Family and friends can offer practical help, such as babysitting, running errands, or providing respite care. This support not only benefits parents but also allows the child to spend time with trusted loved ones.

4. **Celebrating Achievements**: Involve family and friends in celebrating your child's milestones and achievements. Sharing successes with loved ones creates a positive and encouraging environment.

5. **Education and Training**: Family members and friends can participate in education and training

sessions about your child's condition and how they can support their growth and development.

6. **Inclusive Activities**: Plan inclusive activities that involve your child and other family members or friends. Inclusion fosters a sense of belonging and promotes understanding among all family members.

7. **Emotional Support**: Embrace the emotional support offered by loved ones. Talking about your experiences and feelings can strengthen your bond with family and friends.

While involving family and friends can be incredibly beneficial, it is essential to recognize that not everyone may fully grasp the challenges of special needs parenting. Some family members and friends may need time to understand and adjust to the new reality, and that's okay. Providing gentle education and creating opportunities for them to engage with your child can be transformative in their understanding.

In some cases, family members or friends may offer unsolicited advice or make well-intentioned but insensitive comments. It is essential to set boundaries and advocate for our child's needs when necessary. Open communication can play a crucial role in addressing misunderstandings and fostering a supportive environment.

As parents, we must also recognize that family and friends may have their struggles in understanding and accepting the challenges of special needs parenting. Their emotions and concerns are valid, and providing them with resources and support can help them navigate their journey of understanding and support.

In some cases, we may encounter resistance or lack of support from certain family members or friends. It can be disheartening, but it is crucial to focus on those who are supportive and willing to be part of our child's life. Surrounding ourselves and our children with love and positivity creates a nurturing and empowering environment for everyone involved.

In conclusion, building a robust support network is an indispensable aspect of special needs parenting. Engaging with support groups, connecting with other parents, and involving family and friends enriches our lives, provides invaluable resources, and creates a sense of belonging for our children and ourselves.

Together, we form a community of strength, empathy, and understanding that enables us to embrace the challenges and triumphs of special needs parenting with resilience and love. As we weave this tapestry of support around our families, we find solace in the knowledge that we are not alone and that our collective journey is one of beauty, growth, and endless possibilities.

CHAPTER 4

Creating an Inclusive Home Environment

Home is more than just a physical space; it is a sanctuary of love, comfort, and acceptance. For families with children who have special needs, the home becomes an essential foundation for fostering growth, development, and a sense of belonging. Creating an inclusive home environment is about embracing diversity and adapting our living spaces to cater to the unique needs of our children. In this chapter, we explore the art of making our homes accessible, fostering sensory-friendly spaces, and promoting communication and socialization in an environment that celebrates the beauty of individual differences.

4.1   Adapting the Home for Accessibility

In an inclusive home environment, accessibility is a cornerstone. Adapting the home to meet the specific needs of our children creates an empowering space where they can navigate independently and participate fully in family life. The goal is to eliminate physical barriers and create an environment that fosters both independence and safety.

Here are some considerations for adapting the home for accessibility:

1. **Safety Measures**: Ensuring safety is paramount. Installing safety gates, securing furniture, and placing childproof locks on cabinets are essential measures, especially for children with mobility or sensory challenges.

2. **Ramps and Rails:** For children with mobility impairments, installing ramps and handrails can facilitate movement throughout the home. These modifications promote independence and reduce the risk of falls.

3. **Accessible Bathrooms**: Adapting bathrooms with grab bars, non-slip mats, and raised toilet seats can make bathing and using the facilities more manageable for children with physical disabilities.

4. **Sensory Considerations**: Pay attention to lighting, colors, and textures in the home. Soft, natural lighting and calming colors can create a soothing atmosphere while avoiding overly stimulating elements can be beneficial for children with sensory processing challenges.

5. **Organization and Storage**: Keeping the home organized and clutter-free can reduce sensory overload and create a more calming environment for children who are easily overwhelmed.

6. **Visual Supports**: Incorporate visual supports, such as picture schedules and labels, to aid children with communication or cognitive challenges in understanding daily routines and tasks.

7. **Quiet Spaces**: Designating quiet spaces in the home where children can retreat when feeling overwhelmed or overstimulated is essential for promoting self-regulation.

8. **Flexible Furniture Arrangement**: Consider arranging furniture in a way that allows for easy navigation and movement throughout the home, especially for children with mobility aids.

9. **Communication Accessibility**: Implementing accessible communication tools, such as communication boards or devices, ensures that children with communication challenges can express their needs and desires effectively.

10: **Involving Children**: Involve children in the process of adapting the home to meet their needs. This empowers them and fosters a sense of ownership and belonging.

Adapting the home for accessibility is an ongoing process that may require adjustments as the child's needs change over time. Consulting with occupational therapists or accessibility specialists can provide valuable insights and guidance in making appropriate modifications.

It is essential to strike a balance between creating an accessible home and maintaining a warm and welcoming atmosphere. An inclusive home environment celebrates the uniqueness of each family member while fostering a sense of togetherness and belonging.

4.2 Fostering Sensory-Friendly Spaces

For children with sensory processing challenges, the home environment can have a profound impact on their well-being and comfort. Sensory-friendly spaces are designed to minimize sensory overload and create environments where children can explore, learn, and thrive without feeling overwhelmed.

Here are some strategies for fostering sensory-friendly spaces at home:

1. **Calming Colors and Lighting**: Choose soft, neutral colors for walls and furniture to create a calming atmosphere. Natural light is ideal, but when artificial lighting is needed, opt for dimmable, warm-colored lights.

2. **Sensory Diet Stations**: Set up sensory diet stations with various sensory tools, such as weighted blankets, fidget toys, and sensory bins. These stations can provide sensory input that supports self-regulation.

3. **Soft Textures**: Incorporate soft, comfortable textures in furniture, rugs, and bedding to create a soothing environment.

4. **Noise Reduction**: Minimize noise distractions by using noise-canceling curtains, rugs, or white noise machines in sensory-sensitive areas.

5. **Visual Organization**: Keep visual clutter to a minimum to reduce sensory overload. Use storage bins and labels to keep toys and belongings organized.

6. **Cozy Retreats**: Designate cozy nooks or quiet spaces where children can retreat when they need a break from sensory stimulation.

7. **Sensory Play Areas**: Create sensory play areas where children can engage in activities that stimulate their senses in a positive and controlled way.

8. **Individualized Sensory Profiles**: Each child's sensory needs are unique. Observe and understand your child's sensory preferences and aversions to tailor the sensory environment accordingly.

9. **Incorporate Nature**: Nature has a calming effect on the senses. Consider incorporating natural elements such as plants, natural materials, or a small indoor garden into the home.

10. **Sensory Exploration**: Encourage sensory exploration in safe and supervised ways. Engaging in activities like water play, sand play, or finger painting can be beneficial for sensory development.

Remember that sensory-friendly spaces are not about limiting a child's experiences but rather creating an environment where they feel comfortable and supported. A sensory-friendly home fosters self-regulation, emotional well-being, and a sense of security, allowing children to explore the world at their pace.

4.3 Promoting Communication and Socialization

Effective communication and socialization are essential life skills that open doors to meaningful relationships and a sense of belonging. In an inclusive home environment, promoting communication and socialization is about creating opportunities for our children to express themselves, engage with others, and build connections.

Here are some strategies for promoting communication and socialization at home:

1. **Communication-Rich Environment**: Foster a communication-rich environment by engaging in conversations, storytelling, and asking open-ended questions. Encourage children to express their thoughts, feelings, and desires.

2. **Augmentative and Alternative Communication (AAC)**: For children with communication challenges, consider using AAC tools, such as picture communication boards, communication devices, or sign language, to support communication.

3. **Turn-Taking and Listening**: Encourage turn-taking during conversations and activities, emphasizing active listening and respecting each other's perspectives.

4. **Peer Play**: Arrange playdates and activities with peers, siblings, or cousins to promote social interactions and friendships.

5. **Social Stories**: Use social stories or role-play to teach social skills and appropriate behaviors in different situations.

6. **Inclusive Play**: Create opportunities for inclusive play where siblings and friends can engage in activities that accommodate the needs of all children involved.

7. **Social Scripts**: Develop social scripts for common social situations to provide children with guidance on appropriate social responses.

8. **Joint Activities**: Engage in joint activities as a family, such as cooking together, playing board games, or going on outings, to promote bonding and communication.

9. **Emphasize Empathy**: Teach empathy and understanding by discussing feelings and emotions openly and encouraging children to consider others' perspectives.

10. **Visual Schedules**: Use visual schedules to help children understand and anticipate daily routines, transitions, and upcoming events.

11. **Modeling Social Skills**: Model positive social interactions and communication for children to observe and learn from.

12: **Peer Support**: Encourage older siblings or family members to support and engage with their younger siblings in inclusive play.

Promoting communication and socialization is an ongoing process that requires patience, understanding, and consistent effort. It is essential to create an environment where children feel comfortable and confident in expressing themselves and connecting with others. By fostering communication and socialization at home, we empower our children with the tools they need to build meaningful relationships, navigate social situations, and thrive in their interactions with the world around them.

In an inclusive home environment, communication and socialization are not limited to verbal interactions alone. It is essential to recognize and embrace different forms of communication and expressions of socialization. Some children may communicate through gestures, facial expressions, or nonverbal cues, and it is crucial to validate and respond to these unique modes of expression.

Overall, creating an inclusive home environment is a labor of love that involves adaptation, understanding, and unconditional acceptance. It is about embracing the diversity within our families and celebrating the unique gifts and challenges of each child. By adapting the home for accessibility, fostering sensory-friendly spaces, and promoting communication and socialization, we cultivate an environment where our children can flourish and reach their full potential.

An inclusive home is a sanctuary of support, a place where our children can be themselves without judgment or limitation. It is a place where they can explore, learn, and grow, surrounded by love, understanding, and acceptance. As parents, we are the architects of this inclusive home, crafting an environment that nurtures the beautiful tapestry of our family.

As we embark on this journey, let us remember that each child is a shining star, guiding us toward a future of compassion, inclusivity, and boundless possibilities. Together, we create a home that is not just a physical space but a sanctuary of love, where our children can spread their wings and soar beyond the boundaries of expectations and limitations.

In building an inclusive home environment, we also create a ripple effect that extends far beyond our four walls. Our inclusive home becomes a beacon of inspiration for others, showcasing the beauty of diversity and the power of acceptance. As we navigate the highs and lows of special needs parenting, may our homes stand as a testament to the unwavering love and dedication that fuels our journey.

In the spirit of inclusivity, let us reach out to our communities and beyond, sharing our experiences, wisdom, and insights. Together, we can build a world that celebrates the uniqueness of every child, where differences are not just accepted but embraced with open arms.

In the end, an inclusive home environment is not just a physical space—it is a state of mind and a way of living. It is a journey of growth, learning, and transformation that we embark on hand in hand with our children, celebrating their abilities, nurturing their dreams, and empowering them to shine brightly in the world.

As we create an inclusive home, we create a legacy of love and acceptance that will resonate for generations to come. It is a legacy that transcends time and space, reminding us that in the tapestry of life, every thread, no matter how different, is an essential part of the whole.

CHAPTER 5

Nurturing Communication Skills

Communication is the lifeblood of human interaction, the bridge that connects hearts and minds, and the foundation of meaningful relationships. For children with special needs, nurturing communication skills is a transformative journey that empowers them to express their thoughts, emotions, and needs, and fosters a sense of belonging and understanding within their families and communities. In this chapter, we explore the power of alternative communication methods, the art of encouraging language development, and the strategies for building effective communication techniques that embrace the unique communication styles of every child.

5.1 Using Alternative Communication Methods

For some children with special needs, verbal communication may present challenges due to speech delays, language disorders, or other communication impairments. In such cases, alternative communication methods offer a powerful means of expression, giving children a voice and a way to interact with the world.

Alternative communication methods can take various forms, and the key is to find the mode of communication that best suits each child's individual needs and abilities.

Some common alternative communication methods include:

1. **Augmentative and Alternative Communication (AAC)**: AAC encompasses a wide range of tools and strategies that support or replace verbal communication. AAC can include communication boards, picture exchange communication systems (PECS), communication apps, and speech-generating devices. These tools enable children to communicate using symbols, pictures, or written words.

2. **Sign Language**: American Sign Language (ASL) and other sign languages provide a visual means of communication for children with hearing impairments or language delays. Learning sign language can enhance communication and social interactions.

3. **Visual Supports**: Visual supports, such as schedules, choice boards, and visual cues, aid comprehension and facilitate communication for children who benefit from visual prompts.

4. **Gesture and Body Language**: Encouraging and interpreting gestures and body language can be an essential means of communication for some children.

5. **Sensory Communication**: Some children may communicate through sensory responses, such as

pointing, touching, or vocalizing, to express their needs or preferences.

6. **Assistive Technology**: Various assistive technologies, including eye-gaze devices or switches, can empower children with severe physical impairments to communicate effectively.

When introducing alternative communication methods, it is essential to consider each child's communication preferences, motor skills, cognitive abilities, and sensory needs. The goal is to provide a means of communication that is intuitive, efficient, and meaningful for the child.

It is crucial to recognize that using alternative communication methods does not hinder language development but rather supports and enhances it. Alternative communication methods provide a foundation upon which children can build their language skills and participate more actively in conversations and social interactions.

To implement alternative communication methods effectively, involve speech-language pathologists, occupational therapists, and other communication specialists who can assess the child's needs and guide the selection and implementation of appropriate tools and strategies. Collaboration with these professionals ensures that the chosen methods align with the child's goals and facilitate successful communication.

Additionally, involving the entire family and support network in learning and using alternative communication methods creates a consistent and inclusive environment where the child's voice is heard and respected.

5.2   Encouraging   Language Development

For children with special needs who are developing verbal communication skills, fostering language development is a journey of patience, support, and exploration. Encouraging language development involves creating a language-rich environment that supports the child's communication efforts and provides ample opportunities for language exploration and growth.

Here are some strategies for encouraging language development:

1. **Language Modeling**: Model rich and varied language during conversations and interactions with the child. Use descriptive language, expand on their utterances, and introduce new words to enhance vocabulary.

2. **Narration**: Narrate daily activities, routines, and experiences to provide context and support comprehension. Narration can be especially helpful for children with language delays or those who benefit from additional reinforcement.

3. **Read Aloud**: Reading aloud to the child introduces them to the rhythm and structure of language, expands their vocabulary, and stimulates their imagination.

4. **Engage in Conversations**: Engage the child in back-and-forth conversations, even if their responses are limited. Listening attentively and responding to their communication attempts encourages further engagement.

5. **Songs and Rhymes**: Singing songs and reciting rhymes can be a fun and engaging way to promote language development, rhythm, and phonological awareness.

6. **Storytelling**: Encourage the child to tell stories or recount their experiences, using visual supports or drawing to aid their storytelling.

7. **Play and Language**: Incorporate play into language activities, as play provides a natural context for language use and exploration.

8. **Joint Attention**: Engage the child in activities that promote joint attention, where they share a focus on an object or activity with a communication partner.

9. **Imitation**: Encourage imitation of sounds, gestures, and words as a stepping stone towards expressive language.

10. **Patience and Encouragement**: Be patient and supportive as the child develops their language skills. Provide positive reinforcement and celebrate their progress, no matter how small or gradual.

11. **Simplify Language**: Adapt your language to match the child's current level of understanding. Use shorter sentences and clear, concise language to aid comprehension.

12. **Give Choices:** Offer the child choices to encourage decision-making and communication. This empowers them to express their preferences and needs.

13. **Incorporate Interests**: Integrate the child's interests and passions into language activities to increase engagement and motivation.

14. **Multimodal Communication**: Recognize and embrace the child's unique communication style, which may involve a combination of gestures, vocalizations, and other forms of expression.

15. **Playful Interactions**: Engage in playful interactions that invite language exploration, such as pretend play, storytelling, or role-playing.

16. **Create Language-Rich Environments**: Surround the child with language by labeling objects, using visual supports, and incorporating language into daily routines.

17. **Peer Interactions**: Encourage interactions with peers to promote language development through social play and communication.

18. **Recognize Nonverbal Communication**: Acknowledge and respond to the child's nonverbal communication, such as facial expressions and body language, to build trust and understanding.

19: **Be Present and Attentive**: Be fully present and attentive during communication interactions. This shows the child that their communication efforts are valued and respected.

20. **Seek Professional Guidance**: Collaborate with speech-language pathologists and other language specialists to develop an individualized language development plan that addresses the child's unique needs.

Language development is a gradual and dynamic process that unfolds over time. Each child's journey is unique, and progress may occur at different rates. By fostering a language-rich environment and embracing each child's pace, we create an environment that nurtures language development and fosters a positive and empowering experience.

5.3 Building Effective Communication Techniques

Effective communication techniques are the building blocks of successful interactions and meaningful connections. For children with special needs, developing effective communication techniques goes beyond verbal language—it encompasses the use of alternative communication methods, social skills, and emotional regulation.

Here are some strategies for building effective communication techniques:

1. **Active Listening**: Practice active listening by giving the child your full attention, maintaining eye contact, and providing verbal and nonverbal cues that you are engaged and receptive.

2. **Reinforce Communication Attempts**: Encourage and reinforce the child's communication

attempts, whether through words, gestures, or other modes of expression. Responding to their communication signals validation and encourages further communication.

3. **Visual Supports**: Use visual supports, such as visual schedules, choice boards, and communication aids, to enhance comprehension and provide structure during interactions.

4. **Wait Time**: Give the child sufficient wait time to process information and formulate their response. Avoid rushing or interrupting their communication.

5. **Turn-Taking**: Model and encourage turn-taking during conversations and social interactions to promote reciprocal communication.

6. **Social Scripts**: Use social scripts to help the child navigate social situations and practice appropriate social responses.

7. **Social Cues**: Teach the child to recognize and respond to social cues, such as facial expressions, body language, and tone of voice.

8. **Emotional Regulation**: Support the child in developing emotional regulation skills, as emotions can significantly impact communication.

9. **Role-Playing**: Engage in role-playing activities to practice social skills and problem-solving in a safe and supportive environment.

10: **Peer Interactions**: Provide opportunities for the child to interact with peers, promoting social communication and cooperation.

11. **Visual Communication Prompts**: Use visual communication prompts, such as pictures or gestures, to aid understanding and reinforce key concepts during interactions.

12. **Respect Individual Pace**: Be patient and respect the child's pace of communication. Avoid pressure or expectations that may hinder their comfort and confidence in expressing themselves.

13. **Positive Reinforcement**: Provide positive reinforcement for effective communication techniques, praising the child for their efforts and progress.

14. **Flexibility**: Be flexible in communication styles and adapt to the child's preferred mode of communication. Embrace alternative communication methods to meet the child's unique needs.

15. **Collaboration**: Collaborate with educators, therapists, and other support professionals to implement consistent communication strategies across home, school, and other settings.

16. **Use Visual Schedules**: Implement visual schedules and calendars to support understanding and predictability in daily routines.

17: **Provide Choices**: Offer choices to empower the child in decision-making and encourage communication.

18: **Acknowledge Feelings**: Acknowledge and validate the child's feelings, creating a supportive environment for communication.

19: **Mindful Responses**: Be mindful of your responses to the child's communication attempts, ensuring they feel heard and valued.

20. **Create a Communication-Rich Environment**: Foster a communication-rich environment that encourages exploration and practice of communication skills.

Building effective communication techniques is a collaborative effort that involves understanding and embracing the child's unique communication style. It is about creating an environment where the child feels comfortable and empowered to express themselves authentically.

Effective communication techniques extend beyond the child's immediate environment, encompassing interactions with family members, peers, teachers, and the broader community. By fostering effective communication techniques, we equip our children with the tools they need to navigate a world that celebrates their voice and unique communication style.

In conclusion, nurturing communication skills is a transformative journey of connection, empowerment, and growth. By using alternative communication methods, encouraging language development, and building effective communication techniques, we create an inclusive environment where every child's voice is heard, understood, and celebrated.

In the tapestry of communication, every thread, whether verbal, nonverbal, or alternative, is an essential part of the whole. As parents, educators, and caregivers, we are the weavers of this tapestry, creating an environment where communication is not a barrier but a bridge that connects hearts and minds.

As we nurture communication skills, we embrace the beauty of individual differences and celebrate the richness of diverse communication styles. We recognize that effective communication is not a one-size-fits-all approach but a personalized journey that honors each child's unique needs and abilities.

CHAPTER 6

Finding the Right Educational Setting

Education is a transformative journey that lays the foundation for a child's future, shaping their knowledge, skills, and aspirations. For parents of children with special needs, finding the right educational setting is a crucial decision that impacts their child's academic, social, and emotional development. In this chapter, we explore the diverse options available, from inclusive classrooms that celebrate diversity to specialized schools that cater to specific needs and alternative approaches like homeschooling. By understanding the unique benefits and considerations of each setting, parents can make informed choices that best support their child's educational journey.

6.1 Exploring Inclusive Classrooms

Inclusive classrooms embrace diversity and create an environment where children of all abilities learn side by side. Inclusion goes beyond physical presence; it fosters a sense of belonging and encourages active participation and engagement for every student. For children with special needs, inclusion offers numerous benefits, including social interaction, exposure to grade-level curriculum, and opportunities for peer learning.

Key Features of Inclusive Classrooms:

1. **Differentiated Instruction**: Teachers in inclusive classrooms use differentiated instruction to accommodate diverse learning styles and abilities. They tailor teaching strategies, materials, and assessments to meet the needs of each student.

2. **Collaboration**: Inclusi Tove classrooms promote collaboration among teachers, specialists, and support staff. This team approach ensures that every child receives the appropriate accommodations and interventions to succeed academically and socially.

3. **Positive Role Models**: Inclusion allows children with special needs to observe positive role models among their peers. They witness age-appropriate behavior, social interactions, and academic achievements, fostering motivation and self-esteem.

4. **Social Interaction**: Inclusive classrooms provide ample opportunities for social interaction, promoting friendships and reducing the risk of social isolation often experienced by children with special needs in segregated settings.

5. **Access to General Education Curriculum**: Inclusive classrooms offer access to the general education curriculum, allowing children with special

needs to engage with grade-level content and learn alongside their typically developing peers.

6. **Emotional Benefits**: Being part of an inclusive classroom can enhance a child's emotional well-being, as they feel included and accepted within a diverse community of learners.

7. **Increased Empathy**: Inclusive classrooms promote understanding and empathy among students, as they learn to appreciate and respect individual differences.

Factors to Consider:

1. **Teacher Training and Support**: Inclusive classrooms require teachers who are trained in special education and experienced in implementing inclusive practices. Adequate support and professional development are essential to ensure the success of inclusive education.

2. **Individualized Education Plans (IEPs)**: For children with special needs, the development and implementation of IEPs are critical components of inclusion. An effective IEP outlines the child's specific learning goals and necessary accommodations to support their progress.

3. **Classroom Environment**: The physical classroom environment should be organized to accommodate diverse learning needs, providing accessibility and sensory-friendly spaces when required.

4. **Peer Relationships**: Consider the social dynamics of the classroom and how well students with special

needs are integrated into social activities and peer interactions.

5. **Support Services**: Inquire about the availability of support services, such as speech therapy, occupational therapy, or behavior intervention, within the inclusive classroom.

6. **Communication and Collaboration**: Assess how effectively the school fosters communication and collaboration among teachers, parents, and specialists to ensure a cohesive approach to inclusive education.

Inclusive classrooms can be a nurturing and empowering educational setting for children with special needs. The opportunity to learn alongside typically developing peers can offer a well-rounded and enriching experience that celebrates diversity and promotes academic and social growth.

6.2 Considering Specialized Schools

Specialized schools focus on addressing the specific needs of children with particular disabilities or learning challenges. These schools offer a tailored and targeted approach to education, providing a specialized curriculum, therapeutic interventions, and individualized support.

Key Features of Specialized Schools:

1. **Targeted Curriculum**: Specialized schools offer a curriculum that aligns with the unique learning needs of their students. The curriculum may be adapted, modified, or designed specifically for children with certain disabilities.
2. **Therapeutic Services**: Specialized schools often have access to a range of therapeutic services, including speech therapy, occupational therapy, physical therapy, and counseling.
3. **Small Class Sizes**: Class sizes are typically smaller in specialized schools, allowing for more individualized attention and support.
4. **Highly Trained Staff**: Teachers and staff in specialized schools are often trained and experienced in working with children with specific disabilities, offering expertise in addressing their learning challenges.
5. **Focused Environment**: Specialized schools create an environment that is specifically tailored to the needs of the students, providing a supportive and understanding setting.

6.3 Homeschooling and Alternative Approaches

Homeschooling and alternative approaches to education offer flexibility and customization, allowing parents to tailor the learning experience to meet their child's individual needs. Homeschooling can be a viable option for parents who desire more control over their child's education or for children whose needs are best met through a personalized approach.

Key Features of Homeschooling and Alternative Approaches:

1. **Customized Curriculum**: Homeschooling allows parents to design a curriculum that caters to their child's strengths, interests, and learning pace. They can incorporate various teaching methods and resources that align with the child's learning style.

2. **Individualized Attention**: Homeschooling provides one-on-one instruction, allowing parents to focus on their child's specific learning needs and provide immediate feedback and support.

3. **Flexible Schedule**: Homeschooling allows for a flexible schedule, accommodating the child's unique routine, learning preferences, and therapeutic interventions.

4. **Integration of Therapy**: Homeschooling can incorporate therapeutic interventions seamlessly into the child's daily routine, promoting consistency and progress.

5. **Reduced Stress**: Homeschooling can be a less stressful environment for children who may struggle with the social and sensory demands of traditional school settings.

Factors to Consider:

1. Parent's Ability and Commitment: Homeschooling requires a significant commitment of time, effort, and resources from parents or caregivers. It is essential to consider whether the parent has the capacity and willingness to take on the role of an educator.

2. **Access to Resources**: Assess the availability of resources, materials, and support networks for homeschooling in your community.

3. **Socialization Opportunities**: Consider how homeschooling can provide opportunities for social interaction and friendships with peers.

4. **Legal and Regulatory Requirements**: Familiarize yourself with the homeschooling regulations and requirements in your region, as they vary by location.

5. **Transitioning to Future Educational Settings**: Consider how homeschooling may impact the child's transition to future educational settings or post-secondary options.

6. **Balancing Family Dynamics**: Evaluate how homeschooling may impact family dynamics and the roles of other family members.

Alternative approaches to education, such as homeschooling, can be empowering for families seeking a highly personalized and flexible learning experience. By aligning the curriculum and environment with the child's specific needs, parents can create a nurturing educational setting that promotes academic, social, and emotional growth.

Overall, finding the right educational setting for a child with special needs is a deeply personal decision that reflects the family's values, the child's unique strengths, and their specific learning needs. Exploring inclusive classrooms, considering specialized schools, and embracing alternative approaches like homeschooling each offer unique advantages and considerations.

Inclusive classrooms celebrate diversity, foster social interaction, and provide access to grade-level curricula. Specialized schools cater to specific disabilities, offering targeted interventions and therapeutic services. Homeschooling and alternative approaches provide flexibility, customization, and individualized attention, allowing parents to design a curriculum that meets their child's specific needs.

Ultimately, the decision about the right educational setting should be guided by the child's unique strengths, challenges, and learning style. It is essential to consider the child's academic, social, and emotional needs, as well as their overall well-being.

CHAPTER 7

Individualized Education Plans (IEPs) and 504 Plans

Education is a cornerstone of a child's development, and for students with special needs, having a tailored and supportive educational plan is crucial to ensuring academic and overall success. Individualized Education Plans (IEPs) and 504 Plans are essential tools designed to provide personalized support and accommodations for children with disabilities in the educational setting. In this chapter, we delve into the IEP process, the collaboration with school professionals, and the advocacy necessary to secure the best possible plan for your child's unique needs.

7.1 Understanding the IEP Process

An Individualized Education Plan (IEP) is a comprehensive document that outlines the specialized education and related services a child with a disability will receive to support their learning and development. It is a legally binding agreement between the school, parents or guardians, and other relevant stakeholders.

The IEP process involves careful assessment, planning, and implementation, with the ultimate goal of providing the child with the tools they need to thrive academically and socially.

Key Components of an IEP:

1. **Present Levels of Performance**: This section provides a detailed evaluation of the child's current academic and functional performance. It highlights their strengths, challenges, and specific needs in various areas of development.

2. **Measurable Goals and Objectives**: IEPs set clear, measurable, and achievable goals that reflect the child's educational progress and target their areas of improvement. These goals are designed to be specific to the child's needs and align with the curriculum standards.

3. **Accommodations and Modifications**: IEPs include a list of accommodations and modifications that will be provided to support the child's learning. Accommodations are adjustments made to the learning environment or the way information is presented, while modifications involve altering the curriculum or grading criteria.

4. **Related Services**: This section identifies the specialized services the child will receive, such as speech therapy, occupational therapy, counseling, or physical therapy, to address their specific needs.

5. **Transition Planning**: For students approaching graduation or moving to a different school setting,

transition planning outlines the steps and support required to facilitate a smooth transition to post-secondary education or other life endeavors.

6. **Participation in General Education**: IEPs address the child's participation in general education classes and how they will be integrated into the mainstream classroom environment.

7. **Evaluation and Progress Monitoring**: The IEP includes a plan for regularly evaluating the child's progress toward their goals and determining the effectiveness of the interventions and accommodations.

The IEP Team:

The development of an IEP is a collaborative process involving a team of professionals and stakeholders who contribute their expertise and perspectives.

The IEP team typically includes:

1. **Parents or Guardians**: As primary advocates for the child, parents actively participate in the IEP process, sharing their insights, concerns, and goals for their child's education.

2. **General Education Teacher**: The child's general education teacher provides valuable input on their academic performance, classroom behavior, and participation in class activities.

3. **Special Education Teacher**: The special education teacher contributes their expertise in designing and implementing interventions and

accommodations that align with the child's unique needs.

4. **Related Service Providers**: Depending on the child's needs, related service providers such as speech-language pathologists, occupational therapists, or school counselors may be involved in the IEP process.

5. **School Administrator or Principal**: The school administrator ensures that the IEP process is compliant with legal requirements and supports the collaborative effort.

6. **School Psychologist or Assessment Specialist**: These professionals conduct assessments and evaluations to determine the child's present levels of performance and contribute to the development of the IEP goals.

7. **The Child (if appropriate):** Depending on their age and level of maturity, the child may be invited to participate in the IEP meetings, expressing their preferences and aspirations for their education.

7.2 Collaborating with School Professionals

Collaboration between parents and school professionals is essential in developing an effective and impactful IEP. Building a positive and respectful relationship with the IEP team fosters a supportive and open environment for discussing the child's needs, setting goals, and determining appropriate accommodations.

Effective collaboration involves:

1. **Open Communication**: Regular and open communication between parents and school professionals establishes a foundation of trust and understanding. Sharing information about the child's strengths, challenges, and progress helps create a holistic picture of their needs.

2. **Active Participation**: Actively participate in IEP meetings and discussions, advocating for your child's needs and contributing valuable insights about their learning style and preferences.

3. **Listening to Expertise**: Value the expertise of the school professionals, as they bring knowledge and experience in supporting children with disabilities. Be open to their recommendations and suggestions.

4. **Asking Questions**: Don't hesitate to ask questions or seek clarification about the IEP process, goals, or interventions. Understanding every aspect of the plan is essential for effective implementation.

5. **Collaborative Problem-Solving**: Approach challenges as opportunities for collaborative problem-solving. Work together with the IEP team to find solutions that best support the child's learning and development.

6. **Reviewing Progress**: Regularly review the child's progress toward their IEP goals and evaluate the effectiveness of the accommodations and interventions. Discuss adjustments or modifications as needed.

7. **Celebrating Success**: Acknowledge and celebrate the child's achievements and progress, no matter how small. Positive reinforcement and support contribute to the child's motivation and confidence.

Building a positive and collaborative relationship with school professionals not only strengthens the IEP process but also fosters a sense of partnership in supporting the child's education and growth.

7.3 Advocating for Your Child's Needs

As a parent or guardian, advocating for your child's needs is an essential aspect of the IEP process. Advocacy involves being an informed and assertive voice for your child, ensuring that their unique strengths and challenges are recognized and addressed in the IEP.

Effective advocacy includes:

1. **Understanding Your Rights**: Familiarize yourself with the laws and regulations governing special education, including the Individuals with Disabilities Education Act (IDEA) and Section 504 of the Rehabilitation Act. Understanding your rights empowers you to advocate effectively for your child's needs.

2. **Being Informed**: Stay informed about your child's progress, assessment results, and educational options.

Knowledge of your child's strengths and needs will inform your advocacy efforts.

3. **Preparing for IEP Meetings**: Before attending an IEP meeting, review the current IEP, assessments, and progress reports. Prepare a list of questions, concerns, and goals you wish to discuss during the meeting.

4. **Sharing Information**: Share relevant information about your child's medical history, therapies, and any external evaluations or assessments that may impact their learning.

5. **Articulating Your Child's Needs**: Clearly articulate your child's strengths, challenges, and learning preferences during the IEP meetings. Provide specific examples of their behavior, academic progress, and areas that require support.

6. **Requesting Assessments**: If you believe your child's needs are not adequately addressed, request additional assessments or evaluations to gather more comprehensive information about their learning profile.

7. **Collaborating with the IEP Team**: Collaborate with the IEP team in setting appropriate goals and determining suitable interventions and accommodations. Respectfully communicate your opinions and work towards consensus.

8. **Seeking External Support**: If necessary, seek support from special education advocates or organizations that can provide guidance and expertise in the IEP process.

9. **Maintaining Records**: Keep copies of all relevant documents, including evaluations, IEPs, and correspondence related to your child's education. These records can serve as a valuable resource in monitoring your child's progress and advocating for their needs.

10. **Following Up**: After the IEP is developed and implemented, follow up regularly with teachers and school professionals to monitor your child's progress and address any concerns that arise.

11. **Resolving Disputes**: In cases where disagreements arise, be prepared to engage in dispute resolution processes, such as mediation or due process hearings, to ensure your child's needs are met.

12. **Collaborating with Other Parents**: Connect with other parents of children with special needs to share experiences, insights, and resources. Collective advocacy can be a powerful force for positive change.

Remember that advocating for your child's needs is not about confrontation or conflict but about working together with the school to create the best possible educational plan for your child. Emphasize your child's strengths and the unique qualities that make them special while addressing their challenges and learning requirements.

Advocacy is an ongoing process that involves continuous communication, monitoring, and assessment. By being proactive and persistent in advocating for your child, you demonstrate your commitment to their education and well-being.

In conclusion, Individualized Education Plans (IEPs) and 504 Plans are instrumental in ensuring that children with special needs receive the support and accommodations they need to thrive in the educational setting. Understanding the IEP process, collaborating with school professionals, and advocating for your child's needs are essential components of a successful and impactful educational plan.

The IEP process is a collaborative effort involving parents, school professionals, and related service providers. It is a comprehensive and personalized approach to supporting a child's learning and development. By understanding the key components of an IEP and actively participating in the process, parents can play a crucial role in creating a plan that meets their child's unique needs and goals.

Collaborating with school professionals is essential in developing and implementing an effective IEP. Building a positive and respectful relationship with the IEP team fosters an open and supportive environment for discussing the child's needs, setting goals, and determining appropriate accommodations.

Advocating for your child's needs is a vital aspect of the IEP process. As a parent or guardian, you are your child's best advocate, and your knowledge, insights, and assertiveness can make a significant difference in securing the support and resources your child requires.

By understanding the IEP process, collaborating with school professionals, and advocating for your child's needs, you ensure that your child's educational journey empowers and nurtures their unique abilities. With the right support and accommodations in place, every child can reach their full potential, contributing their gifts and talents to the world and embracing a future filled with possibilities.

CHAPTER 8

Supporting Learning at Home

The home is a powerful and nurturing space where a child's love for learning can flourish. For children with special needs, a supportive learning environment at home can play a pivotal role in complementing their education and fostering continuous growth. In this chapter, we explore strategies for creating a structured learning environment, implementing educational activities, and encouraging independence and self-learning to enrich your child's educational journey.

8.1 Creating a Structured Learning Environment

A structured learning environment at home provides a sense of stability, routine, and organization that supports a child's learning and emotional well-being. For children with special needs, the structure is particularly beneficial, as it provides predictability and reduces anxiety. Creating a conducive learning space involves a thoughtful blend of organization, consistency, and adaptability.

Key Elements of a Structured Learning Environment:

1. **Designated Learning Area**: Set aside a specific area in the home for learning activities. This space should be quiet, free from distractions, and well-equipped with educational materials and supplies.

2. **Visual Schedules**: Use visual schedules or calendars to outline daily routines and learning activities. Visual cues provide clarity and predictability for the child.

3. **Consistent Schedule**: Establish a consistent daily or weekly schedule for learning activities. Consistency fosters a sense of routine and helps the child know what to expect each day.

4. **Clear Expectations**: Communicate clear expectations for learning activities and behavior. Encourage the child to take ownership of their learning and progress.

5. **Organizational Systems**: Implement organizational systems for educational materials, books, and resources. Having a designated place for everything promotes efficiency and minimizes distractions.

6. **Sensory-Friendly Environment**: Consider the child's sensory needs when designing the learning space. Create a sensory-friendly environment that supports their comfort and focus.

7. **Positive Reinforcement**: Use positive reinforcement to acknowledge and celebrate the child's efforts and achievements. Encouragement and praise enhance motivation and confidence.

8. **Flexibility**: While structure is essential, allow for flexibility in the learning environment. Adapt the schedule and activities as needed to accommodate the child's unique needs and interests.

8.2   Implementing   Educational Activities

Engaging in educational activities at home not only reinforces learning but also provides opportunities for bonding and shared experiences. Tailor activities to align with the child's interests and learning goals, making learning enjoyable and rewarding.

Ideas for Educational Activities:

1. **Reading Time**: Set aside daily reading time, where you read together or encourage independent reading. Explore books that align with the child's interests and reading level.

2. **Educational Games**: Incorporate educational games and puzzles that promote problem-solving, critical thinking, and creativity.

3. **Hands-On Learning**: Engage in hands-on learning activities, such as science experiments, arts and crafts, or cooking projects. Hands-on activities enhance understanding and retention of concepts.

4. **Learning Apps and Websites**: Utilize educational apps and websites that cater to the child's specific needs and academic goals.

5. **Writing Practice**: Encourage writing practice through journaling, creative writing, or writing letters to family members or friends.

6. **Math Practice**: Integrate math practice into everyday activities, such as counting objects, measuring ingredients, or budgeting for purchases.

7. **Virtual Field Trips**: Take virtual field trips to museums, historical sites, or natural landmarks to explore new subjects and cultures.

8. **Music and Movement**: Incorporate music and movement activities, such as dancing, singing, or playing musical instruments. Music enhances cognitive development and creativity.

9. **STEM Projects**: Engage in science, technology, engineering, and math (STEM) projects that stimulate curiosity and problem-solving skills.

10. **Nature Exploration**: Spend time outdoors exploring nature and observing plants, animals, and natural phenomena.

11. **Learning Through Play**: Integrate learning into play activities, using toys and games to teach new concepts and skills.

12: **Multi-Sensory Activities**: Utilize multi-sensory activities that engage different senses, promoting a holistic learning experience.

8.3 Encouraging Independence and Self-Learning

Fostering independence and self-learning empowers the child to take ownership of their education and fosters a love for learning that extends beyond the confines of formal instruction.

Strategies for Encouraging Independence and Self-Learning:

1. **Choice and Autonomy**: Offer the child choices in their learning activities, allowing them to select topics of interest or the sequence of tasks.

2. **Goal Setting**: Encourage the child to set their learning goals and track their progress. Celebrate achievements and discuss strategies to overcome challenges.

3. **Inquiry-Based Learning**: Encourage curiosity and inquiry-based learning, where the child investigates topics of interest and seeks answers to their questions.

4. **Reflection**: Encourage the child to reflect on their learning experiences, identifying what they enjoyed, what they found challenging, and what they would like to explore further.

5. **Problem-Solving**: Encourage the child to independently solve problems they encounter during

learning activities. Provide guidance when needed but allow space for them to develop problem-solving skills.

5. **Mindfulness and Self-Regulation**: Teach mindfulness techniques and self-regulation strategies to help the child manage stress and emotions during learning.

6. **Peer Learning**: Facilitate opportunities for peer learning and collaborative activities, where the child can share knowledge and learn from others.

7. **Real-World Connections**: Help the child see the real-world applications of what they are learning, making connections between academic concepts and everyday life.

8. **Embrace Mistakes**: Create a safe and supportive environment where mistakes are seen as learning opportunities rather than failures.

9. **Lifelong Learning Mentality**: Model a lifelong learning mentality by demonstrating curiosity, enthusiasm for learning, and continuous personal growth.

Supporting independence and self-learning not only equips the child with valuable skills for their education but also instills a sense of agency and empowerment that will benefit them throughout their lives.

In conclusion, supporting learning at home is a transformative journey that deepens the child's educational experience and nurtures their love for learning. Creating a structured learning environment, implementing educational activities, and encouraging independence and self-learning form the pillars of a supportive home-based education.

By establishing a structured learning environment, parents provide a stable and predictable space where the child can thrive academically and emotionally. A structured environment reduces anxiety and fosters a sense of routine, benefiting children with special needs who often thrive on predictability.

Implementing educational activities at home fosters a love for learning and enhances the child's understanding of academic concepts. Engaging in diverse and enjoyable activities allows children to explore their interests, develop new skills, and expand their knowledge beyond formal education settings.

Encouraging independence and self-learning empowers the child to take ownership of their education and fosters a lifelong love for learning. By encouraging curiosity, choice, and reflection, parents instill in their children a deep sense of agency and a belief in their abilities to navigate the world of knowledge and exploration.

In nurturing learning at home, parents become active partners in their child's education, creating an environment where every child's unique abilities are celebrated and supported. Through the combined efforts of teachers, school professionals, and parents, children with special needs embark on a transformative educational journey filled with growth, discovery, and endless possibilities.

CHAPTER 9

Prioritizing Health and Wellness

As parents of children with special needs, prioritizing health and wellness is essential to ensure their overall well-being and quality of life. Managing medical appointments, promoting healthy habits, and addressing mental and emotional health are crucial aspects of providing comprehensive care for your child. In this chapter, we will explore strategies to effectively prioritize health and wellness, supporting your child's physical, emotional, and mental health needs.

9.1 Managing Medical Appointments

Regular medical appointments are vital for monitoring your child's health, tracking their developmental progress, and addressing any medical concerns promptly. Coordinating and managing medical appointments can be challenging, but it is a critical aspect of providing comprehensive care for your child with special needs.

Strategies for Managing Medical Appointments:

1. **Create a Calendar**: Maintain a detailed calendar to keep track of upcoming medical appointments, therapy sessions, and consultations. Use reminders or digital tools to ensure you don't miss important dates.

2. **Organize Medical Records**: Keep all medical records, test results, and reports organized in a dedicated folder or digital file. This helps you access important information quickly during appointments.

3. **Communicate with Healthcare Providers**: Establish open communication with your child's healthcare providers. Share any changes or concerns regarding your child's health to ensure their care plan remains up-to-date.

4. **Prepare for Appointments**: Before each appointment, write down any questions or concerns you have for the healthcare provider. Being prepared helps make the most of the appointment time.

5. **Involve Your Child**: Depending on their age and understanding, involve your child in discussions about their health and medical care. This helps them feel empowered and engaged in their well-being.

6. **Seek Support**: If managing medical appointments becomes overwhelming, consider seeking support from a care coordinator, social worker, or support group to assist you in navigating the process.

7. **Regular Health Checkups**: In addition to specialized appointments, ensure your child receives regular health checkups with their pediatrician or primary care provider.

Managing medical appointments with diligence and organization allows you to stay on top of your child's health needs and ensures they receive timely and appropriate care.

9.2 Promoting Healthy Habits

Promoting healthy habits is vital for the overall well-being of your child. Healthy lifestyle choices contribute to better physical health, improved cognitive function, and enhanced emotional resilience. As parents, you can play a significant role in fostering healthy habits in your child's daily life.

Strategies for Promoting Healthy Habits:

1. **Balanced Diet**: Encourage a balanced and nutritious diet that includes a variety of fruits, vegetables, whole grains, and lean proteins. Limit the consumption of processed foods and sugary beverages.

2. **Regular Exercise**: Incorporate regular physical activity into your child's daily routine. Adapt activities to their abilities and interests, and engage in exercises that promote strength, flexibility, and cardiovascular health.

3. **Adequate Sleep**: Ensure your child gets enough sleep according to their age and individual needs. A well-rested body supports overall health and contributes to better focus and emotional regulation.

4. **Hygiene Practices**: Teach and reinforce good hygiene practices, such as regular handwashing, dental care, and personal grooming.

5. **Mindful Screen Time**: Monitor and limit screen time, encouraging activities that foster social interaction, creativity, and physical movement.

6. **Family Meals**: Make family meals a regular occurrence, as they provide an opportunity for connection and conversation while promoting healthy eating habits.

7. **Role Model Healthy Behavior**: Model healthy habits yourself, as children often learn by observing their parents' actions.

8. **Stay Hydrated**: Encourage your child to drink plenty of water throughout the day to stay hydrated and support optimal bodily functions.

9. **Outdoor Time**: Spend time outdoors regularly, enjoying nature and engaging in physical activities in the fresh air.

Promoting healthy habits sets the foundation for your child's lifelong well-being. By instilling these habits early on, you equip them with the tools to make positive choices and lead a healthy and fulfilling life.

9.3 Addressing Mental and Emotional Health

Mental and emotional health are integral components of your child's overall well-being. Children with special needs may experience unique challenges related to their emotional development, making it essential to address their mental health with sensitivity and understanding.

Strategies for Addressing Mental and Emotional Health:

1. **Open Communication**: Create an environment of open communication where your child feels comfortable expressing their thoughts and emotions. Encourage them to share their feelings and listen with empathy and support.

2. **Emotional Regulation**: Teach your child strategies for emotional regulation, such as deep breathing, mindfulness techniques, or engaging in calming activities when they feel overwhelmed.

3. **Supportive Environment**: Foster a supportive and nurturing home environment where your child feels safe and loved. Provide emotional support during difficult times and celebrate their achievements.

4. **Social Interaction**: Facilitate opportunities for social interaction with peers and family members. Positive social connections contribute to emotional well-being.

5. **Professional Support**: If needed, seek the support of mental health professionals who have experience working with children with special needs. They can provide valuable guidance and interventions tailored to your child's needs.

6. **Encourage Hobbies and Interests**: Engaging in hobbies and activities your child enjoys can provide a

sense of purpose and fulfillment, positively impacting their emotional well-being.

7. **Mindful Parenting**: Practice mindful parenting, staying attuned to your child's needs and emotions, and responding with patience and understanding.

8. **Sensory Considerations**: Be mindful of your child's sensory needs and how different environments or experiences may impact their emotional well-being.

9. **Normalize Emotions**: Normalize a range of emotions and help your child understand that it's okay to experience different feelings. Encourage open discussions about emotions without judgment.

10. **Monitor Stress Levels**: Be attentive to signs of stress or anxiety in your child and take steps to reduce stressors when possible.

Prioritizing your child's mental and emotional health is as crucial as their physical health. A strong support system and a nurturing approach can help your child navigate emotional challenges and develop resilience in the face of adversity.

Overall, prioritizing health and wellness is a multifaceted journey that encompasses managing medical appointments, promoting healthy habits, and addressing mental and emotional health. As parents, your dedication and support play a central role in ensuring your child's overall well-being and happiness.

By managing medical appointments with diligence and organization, you ensure your child receives the necessary care and support for their unique needs. Promoting healthy habits fosters a strong foundation for their physical health and sets the stage for a lifetime of positive choices.

Addressing your child's mental and emotional health with sensitivity and understanding nurtures their emotional well-being and resilience. By creating a nurturing and supportive environment, you empower your child to thrive emotionally, academically, and socially.

In the tapestry of health and wellness, every thread is vital. With your unwavering dedication and love, your child can embrace a future filled with health, happiness, and a strong sense of well-being.

CHAPTER 10

Sensory Integration and Regulation

For children with special needs, the world can be a sensory-rich environment, presenting both opportunities and challenges in processing sensory information. Sensory integration and regulation are critical aspects of your child's development, impacting their ability to interact with the world around them and engage in daily activities. In this chapter, we will explore the importance of understanding sensory processing, developing sensory integration strategies, and supporting your child's self-regulation skills.

10.1　Understanding Sensory Processing

Sensory processing refers to the way our nervous system interprets and responds to sensory information from the environment. For children with special needs, sensory processing may be atypical, leading to difficulties in effectively processing and responding to sensory stimuli. This can manifest in various ways, such as sensory seeking, sensory sensitivity, or sensory avoidance.

Key Sensory Processing Areas:

1. **Visual**: How the child processes and responds to visual information, such as lights, colors, and patterns.
2. **Auditory**: How the child processes and responds to auditory information, such as sounds, voices, and environmental noises.
3. **Tactile**: How the child processes and responds to tactile information, such as touch, textures, and clothing.
4. **Proprioceptive**: How the child processes and responds to proprioceptive information, relating to body awareness and movement.
5. **Vestibular**: How the child processes and responds to vestibular information, involving balance and movement.

Understanding your child's sensory processing patterns is essential in tailoring strategies to meet their specific sensory needs and support their overall development.

10.2 Developing Sensory Integration Strategies

Sensory integration strategies are designed to help your child effectively process and respond to sensory information, promoting a balanced and regulated sensory experience. These strategies can be incorporated into daily routines and activities to create a sensory-friendly environment.

Sensory Integration Strategies:

1. **Sensory Diet**: Develop a sensory diet in collaboration with occupational therapists. A sensory diet is a personalized plan that includes specific sensory activities to help your child stay regulated and focused.

2. **Sensory Breaks**: Allow your child to take sensory breaks when feeling overwhelmed. These breaks can include activities such as deep breathing exercises, stretching, or spending time in a quiet, calming space.

3. **Calming Sensory Activities**: Introduce calming sensory activities, such as using a weighted blanket, engaging in deep-pressure activities, or playing with sensory toys.

4. **Sensory-Friendly Spaces**: Create sensory-friendly spaces in your home where your child can retreat when feeling overstimulated. These spaces should be quiet, comfortable, and equipped with sensory tools.

5. **Visual Supports**: Use visual supports, such as visual schedules and cues, to help your child navigate daily routines and transitions more smoothly.

6. **Gradual Exposure**: When introducing new sensory experiences, do so gradually to avoid overwhelming your child. Start with gentle exposure and gradually increase the intensity as they become more comfortable.

7. **Sensory Play**: Encourage sensory play activities that engage multiple senses, such as playing with sand, water, or sensory bins.

8. **Fidget Tools**: Provide fidget tools or toys that allow your child to channel excess energy or seek sensory input in a constructive way.

9. **Mindfulness and Sensory Awareness**: Practice mindfulness exercises with your child to enhance their sensory awareness and promote self-regulation.

10. **Communication and Validation**: Encourage open communication with your child about their sensory experiences. Validate their feelings and provide reassurance during challenging sensory moments.

Developing sensory integration strategies tailored to your child's unique sensory profile empowers them to navigate the world with greater ease and confidence.

10.3 Supporting Self-Regulation Skills

Self-regulation is the ability to manage one's emotions, behavior, and responses to the environment effectively. For children with special needs, self-regulation skills are especially important as they can help them cope with sensory challenges and navigate social interactions.

Strategies for Supporting Self-Regulation Skills:

1. **Emotional Awareness**: Help your child recognize and identify their emotions. Use emotion words to label feelings and encourage them to express their emotions verbally.

2. **Coping Strategies**: Teach your child various coping strategies for managing stress and overwhelming emotions. These can include deep breathing, counting to ten, or using a calming tool.

3. **Social Stories**: Use social stories to help your child understand social situations and appropriate responses. Social stories can be valuable tools for teaching self-regulation in different contexts.

4. **Model Self-Regulation**: Model self-regulation techniques yourself. Children often learn best by observing the behavior of adults around them.

5. **Positive Reinforcement**: Provide positive reinforcement and praise when your child demonstrates self-regulation skills, reinforcing their efforts.

6. **Time and Space**: Give your child time and space to self-regulate when needed. Avoid demanding immediate responses during moments of sensory overwhelm.

7. **Sensory Coping Strategies**: Integrate sensory coping strategies into their self-regulation toolkit, such as using sensory tools or engaging in sensory-friendly activities.

8. **Establish Routines**: Routines can provide a sense of predictability and security, supporting your child's ability to self-regulate.

9. **Sensory Awareness**: Help your child become more aware of their sensory experiences and how they affect their emotions and behavior.

10. **Emotional Regulation Games**: Engage in emotional regulation games or activities that make learning self-regulation skills enjoyable and interactive.

By actively supporting your child's self-regulation skills, you empower them to manage their emotions effectively and navigate sensory challenges with greater confidence and resilience.

In conclusion, sensory integration and regulation are fundamental aspects of your child's development and well-being. Understanding their sensory processing patterns, developing sensory integration strategies, and supporting their self-regulation skills are instrumental in nurturing their sensory experiences and fostering their growth.

By acknowledging and addressing your child's unique sensory needs, you provide a nurturing and supportive environment that empowers them to thrive. Sensory integration strategies and self-regulation skills lay the groundwork for your child to engage confidently with the world, manage their emotions effectively, and navigate sensory experiences with greater ease.

As parents and caregivers, your knowledge, empathy, and dedication play a vital role in helping your child embrace their sensory journey with confidence and joy. By incorporating sensory-friendly practices into your child's daily life, you create a space where they can flourish, explore, and reach their full potential in all areas of development.

Chapter 11: Encouraging Physical Activity and Recreation

Physical activity and recreation are essential components of a healthy and fulfilling life for individuals of all abilities, including children with special needs. Engaging in physical activities not only promotes physical well-being but also supports emotional, social, and cognitive development. In this chapter, we will explore ways to encourage physical activity and recreation for children with special needs, finding suitable activities, adapting sports and games, and embracing the joy of play.

11.1 Finding Suitable Activities

When it comes to physical activity, every child is unique, and finding suitable activities that cater to their interests and abilities is key to fostering a positive experience. Consider your child's preferences, strengths, and challenges when exploring different activities.

Strategies for Finding Suitable Activities:

1. **Explore Interests**: Identify activities that align with your child's interests and passions. Whether it's dancing, swimming, biking, or any other activity, finding something they love will enhance their motivation to participate.

2. **Consider Abilities**: Focus on activities that match your child's physical abilities and developmental level. Start with activities that provide a sense of accomplishment and gradually introduce new challenges.

3. **Adaptability**: Look for activities that can be adapted to accommodate your child's unique needs. Many community programs and sports organizations offer inclusive options or are willing to make accommodations.

4. **Consult Therapists**: Consult with your child's therapists or healthcare providers for recommendations on suitable physical activities that align with their therapeutic goals.

5. **Group Activities**: Consider group activities or team sports to provide opportunities for social interaction and peer engagement.

6. **Family Involvement**: Participate in physical activities as a family to make it a fun and bonding experience for everyone.

7. **Age-Appropriate**: Choose activities that are age-appropriate and offer the right level of challenge for your child's age group.

8. **Trial and Error**: Be open to trying different activities to see what resonates best with your child. Don't be discouraged if an activity doesn't work out; there are many options to explore.

Finding suitable activities is a wonderful way to introduce your child to the joy of movement and exploration, supporting their physical development and overall well-being.

11.2 Adapting Sports and Games

Adapting sports and games allows children with special needs to participate fully and enjoy the benefits of physical activity. Simple modifications can make a significant difference in creating an inclusive and supportive environment for all participants.

Strategies for Adapting Sports and Games:

1. **Modify Rules**: Adapt the rules of sports or games to accommodate your child's abilities. For example, in a basketball game, lower the hoop's height or allow more time to complete a task.

2. **Provide Assistive Devices**: Utilize assistive devices or adaptive equipment that support your child's engagement in physical activities. This could include adaptive bikes, wheelchairs, or specialized sporting equipment.

3. **Team Support**: Ensure coaches, teammates, and peers are aware of your child's needs and provide a supportive and inclusive environment.

4. **Individualized Approach**: Focus on your child's progress and individual achievements rather than comparing them to others. Celebrate their efforts and successes, no matter how small.

5. **Create Adaptive Games**: Design adaptive games that cater to your child's specific abilities and interests. Be creative and explore new ways to engage in physical play.

6. **Use Visual Supports**: Use visual cues or pictorial guides to help your child understand game instructions and rules.

7. **Sensory Considerations**: Take sensory needs into account when adapting activities. Create sensory-friendly spaces if needed and be mindful of sensory sensitivities.

8. **Encourage Peer Interaction**: Foster peer interactions and cooperation during sports and games. Encourage inclusive play and teamwork.

Adapting sports and games opens doors to participation and fosters a sense of belonging and achievement for children with special needs. It promotes a positive and empowering experience, encouraging them to embrace physical activity as an enjoyable part of their daily lives.

11.3 Embracing the Joy of Play

Play is a powerful medium for children to learn, explore, and express themselves. Embrace the joy of playing with your child, allowing them the freedom to be themselves and encouraging their natural curiosity and creativity.

Strategies for Embracing the Joy of Play:

1. **Unstructured Playtime**: Offer unstructured playtime where your child can explore freely and use their imagination without constraints.

2. **Playful Activities**: Integrate playfulness into daily routines and activities, turning tasks into enjoyable games.

3. **Sensory Play**: Encourage sensory play activities that engage different senses, providing a rich and stimulating experience.

4. **Playdates and Social Play**: Organize playdates with peers or siblings to foster social interaction and peer play.

5. **Model Playfulness**: Model playfulness yourself, demonstrating enthusiasm and enjoyment in shared activities.

6. **Outdoor Exploration**: Spend time outdoors, allowing your child to connect with nature and engage in physical play.

7. **Art and Creativity**: Encourage artistic expression and creativity through art activities, music, and storytelling.

8. **Play-Based Learning**: Integrate play-based learning into your child's educational journey, making learning enjoyable and engaging.

Embracing the joy of play allows your child to experience the world with wonder and curiosity. Through play, they can build essential life skills, develop social connections, and express their thoughts and emotions.

Overall, encouraging physical activity and recreation is a wonderful way to support your child's development, health, and well-being. Finding suitable activities that align with their interests and abilities, adapting sports and games to create inclusive environments, and embracing the joy of play all contribute to a positive and enriching experience for children with special needs.

By creating a supportive and playful atmosphere, you empower your child to explore, grow, and develop their physical skills with confidence. Remember that each child's journey is unique, and the most meaningful outcomes often arise from nurturing their individual passions and abilities.

Through physical activity and recreation, your child can thrive, discover their strengths, and experience the joy of movement and exploration. With your love, support, and encouragement, they can embrace a lifetime of active living and joyful play.

CHAPTER 12

Transitioning to Adulthood

The transition from adolescence to adulthood is a significant milestone for individuals with special needs and their families. This period brings new opportunities and challenges as young adults embark on their journey toward independence and self-determination. In this chapter, we will explore essential aspects of transitioning to adulthood, including preparing for post-secondary education, exploring vocational opportunities, and navigating the path to independent living.

12.1 Preparing for Post-Secondary Education

For many young adults, pursuing post-secondary education is a valuable pathway to personal and professional growth. Preparing for this transition requires careful planning, collaboration, and a clear understanding of the available resources and support.

Strategies for Preparing for Post-Secondary Education:

1. **Early Planning**: Start planning for post-secondary education during the high school years. Work with school counselors and educators to outline academic goals and discuss potential educational opportunities.

2. **Research Educational Options**: Explore different post-secondary education options, including universities, colleges, vocational schools, and online courses. Consider programs that offer inclusive and accommodating learning environments.

3. **Seek Support Services**: Research the support services available for students with special needs at different educational institutions. Look into disability support offices, counseling services, and academic accommodations.

4. **Visit Campuses**: Schedule campus visits to get a sense of the atmosphere and support available. Encourage your young adult to ask questions and participate in campus tours or open houses.

5. **Individualized Education Plans (IEPs):** Review your child's IEP to identify transition goals and any necessary accommodations for their post-secondary education.

6. **Self-Advocacy Skills**: Foster self-advocacy skills in your young adult, empowering them to communicate their needs and seek support when required.

7. **Financial Planning**: Explore financial aid options and scholarships available for students with disabilities. Create a budget to manage educational expenses.

8. **Mentorship and Guidance**: Connect with mentors or individuals who have experienced a similar transition. Seek guidance from support organizations that specialize in post-secondary education for individuals with special needs.

Preparing for post-secondary education involves a collaborative effort between the young adult, their family, educators, and support professionals. By laying a strong foundation for their educational journey, you set the stage for a fulfilling and successful transition to adulthood.

12.2 Exploring Vocational Opportunities

For some young adults, pursuing vocational opportunities provides a pathway to meaningful employment and personal fulfillment. Vocational training and job exploration offer valuable experiences that help individuals discover their interests and strengths.

Strategies for Exploring Vocational Opportunities:

1. **Vocational Assessment**: Consider vocational assessments to identify your young adult's interests, aptitudes, and potential career paths.
2. **Job Shadowing**: Arrange job shadowing opportunities to expose your young adult to various work environments and professions.
3. **Vocational Training Programs**: Explore vocational training programs that provide hands-on experience and skills development in specific industries.
4. **Supported Employment**: Investigate supported employment programs that offer job coaching and ongoing support in the workplace.
5. **Volunteer Work**: Encourage your young adult to engage in volunteer work, which can provide valuable experience and build their resume.
6. **Career Counseling**: Seek career counseling services to help your young adult set vocational goals and create a plan for achieving them.
7. **Networking**: Build a network of contacts within industries of interest. Networking can lead to job opportunities and mentorship.
8. **Flexibility and Exploration**: Be open to exploring different vocational opportunities. Sometimes the most unexpected paths can lead to fulfilling careers.

Exploring vocational opportunities allows young adults to discover their passions and strengths, leading to a sense of purpose and achievement in their professional lives.

12.3 Navigating Independent Living

As young adults transition to adulthood, navigating the path to independent living becomes a crucial aspect of their journey. Developing life skills, fostering self-reliance, and building a support network are essential for a successful transition.

Strategies for Navigating Independent Living:

1. **Life Skills Training**: Teach essential life skills, such as cooking, cleaning, budgeting, and personal care. Focus on building skills that promote independence and self-sufficiency.

2. **Supported Living Programs**: Research supported living programs that offer assistance and guidance for young adults with special needs as they transition to living independently.

3. **Roommates or Housemates**: Consider living arrangements with roommates or housemates who share similar interests and values.

4. **Transportation Independence**: Encourage your young adult to learn how to use public transportation or

explore other transportation options for increased mobility.

5. **Community Involvement**: Engage in community activities and events to foster a sense of belonging and social interaction.

6. **Emergency Preparedness**: Teach your young adult about emergency preparedness and how to handle unexpected situations.

7. **Legal and Financial Planning**: Investigate legal and financial options to ensure your young adult's rights and financial security are protected.

8. **Support Network**: Build a support network of friends, family, and professionals who can offer guidance and assistance as needed.

Navigating independent living is a transformative process that requires patience, guidance, and flexibility. By nurturing your young adult's independence and self-reliance, you empower them to lead fulfilling and autonomous lives.

In conclusion, transitioning to adulthood is a significant and transformative journey for young adults with special needs. Preparing for post-secondary education, exploring vocational opportunities, and navigating the path to independent living are crucial aspects of this transition.

By fostering a supportive and empowering environment, you enable your young adult to pursue their aspirations and embrace the next chapter of their lives with confidence and enthusiasm. Through careful planning, collaboration, and a commitment to lifelong learning, you empower them to thrive as independent, capable, and fulfilled adults. With your unwavering support and encouragement, they can embark on a journey filled with opportunities, personal growth, and meaningful experiences.

CHAPTER 13

Legal and Financial Considerations

Navigating the legal and financial aspects of caring for a loved one with special needs requires careful consideration and proactive planning. Understanding disability rights, planning for financial security, and accessing government assistance programs are crucial steps in ensuring your family's well-being and protecting the rights of your loved one. In this chapter, we will explore key legal and financial considerations for families with special needs.

13.1 Understanding Disability Rights

Knowing and advocating for disability rights is essential in ensuring that individuals with special needs have equal opportunities and access to the support they need. Familiarize yourself with relevant laws and regulations to ensure that your loved one's rights are protected and respected.

Key Aspects of Disability Rights:

1. **Americans with Disabilities Act (ADA):** Familiarize yourself with the ADA, which prohibits discrimination against individuals with disabilities in areas such as employment, public accommodations, transportation, and telecommunications.

2. **Individuals with Disabilities Education Act (IDEA):** Understand the provisions of IDEA, which guarantees a free appropriate public education (FAPE) to children with disabilities and outlines their rights in the education system.

3. **Housing Rights**: Be aware of housing rights and reasonable accommodations for individuals with disabilities in rental housing or home ownership.

4. **Healthcare Rights**: Understand your loved one's rights in the healthcare system, including access to medical care, accommodations, and patient privacy.

5. **Social Security Disability Insurance (SSDI) and Supplemental Security Income (SSI):** Learn about these federal programs that provide financial support to individuals with disabilities.

6. **Decision-Making Rights**: Be aware of guardianship and alternative decision-making options for adults with special needs who may require assistance in managing their affairs.

7. **Voting Rights**: Ensure that your loved one's right to vote is protected, and they have access to accessible voting options.

Understanding disability rights empowers you to advocate effectively for your loved one's needs and ensures they receive the support and accommodations they are entitled to under the law.

13.2 Planning for Financial Security

Financial planning is a critical aspect of providing for the future well-being of individuals with special needs. Planning for financial security involves creating a comprehensive plan that addresses their long-term needs and safeguards their financial future.

Strategies for Financial Planning:

1. **Special Needs Trust**: Consider establishing a special needs trust, which allows you to set aside funds for your loved one's benefit without affecting their eligibility for government assistance programs.

2. **Financial Advisor**: Consult a financial advisor experienced in special needs planning to help you create a customized plan that aligns with your family's goals and resources.

3. **Life Insurance**: Evaluate the need for life insurance to provide financial protection for your loved one in case of unexpected circumstances.

4. **Government Benefits**: Familiarize yourself with the impact of government benefits on your loved one's financial planning and eligibility.

5. **Employment and Vocational Training**: Explore employment opportunities and vocational training programs that can contribute to your loved one's financial independence.

6. **Public and Private Assistance**: Research public and private assistance programs that can support your family's financial needs and enhance the quality of life for your loved one.

7. **Estate Planning**: Develop a comprehensive estate plan that includes wills, healthcare directives, and guardianship arrangements, ensuring that your loved one's future is secure.

8. **Regular Review**: Regularly review and update your financial plan to adapt to changing circumstances and needs.

Financial planning provides peace of mind and a solid foundation for your loved one's future, ensuring that they can access the resources they need to thrive.

13.3 Accessing Government Assistance Programs

Government assistance programs offer vital support and resources to individuals with special needs and their families. Understanding and accessing these programs can significantly enhance your loved one's quality of life and ease the financial burden.

Key Government Assistance Programs:

1. **Social Security Disability Insurance (SSDI):** Provides financial assistance to individuals with disabilities who have contributed to the Social Security system through their work history.
Supplemental Security Income (SSI): Offers financial support to individuals with disabilities with limited income and resources.
2. **Medicaid:** Provides healthcare coverage to individuals with low income, including those with disabilities.
3. **Medicare**: Offers healthcare coverage to individuals aged 65 and older and to some individuals with disabilities.
4. **Developmental Disabilities (DD) Services**: State-funded programs that offer a range of services and support to individuals with developmental disabilities.
Vocational Rehabilitation (VR) Services: Assists individuals with disabilities in accessing vocational training, employment services, and job placement.
Housing Assistance: Various housing assistance programs provide affordable housing options for individuals with disabilities.
Education Services: Access resources and support available through the Individuals with Disabilities Education Act (IDEA) to ensure your loved one receives appropriate educational services.

Navigating government assistance programs may involve complex processes and eligibility criteria. Work with professionals, such as social workers or disability advocates, to help you navigate the application and qualification process effectively.

Overall, legal and financial considerations are vital aspects of caring for individuals with special needs. Understanding disability rights allows you to advocate effectively and ensure equal opportunities for your loved one. Planning for financial security provides peace of mind and a secure future. Accessing government assistance programs offers essential support and resources to enhance your loved one's quality of life.

By proactively addressing legal and financial considerations, you safeguard your loved one's rights and create a strong foundation for their long-term well-being. Collaboration with professionals and support organizations can provide valuable guidance in navigating these complex areas, ensuring that your family's journey is guided by knowledge, empowerment, and advocacy. With thoughtful planning and advocacy, you create a pathway toward a bright and secure future for your loved one with special needs.

CHAPTER 14

Embracing Change and Celebrating Successes

The journey of special needs parenting is a dynamic and ever-changing path, filled with both challenges and triumphs. Embracing change, celebrating milestones and achievements, and fostering resilience are essential components of navigating this extraordinary journey with grace and strength. In this final chapter, we will explore the importance of embracing the ups and downs, finding joy in celebrating successes and nurturing resilience in both parent and child.

14.1 Embracing the Journey's Ups and Downs

The journey of special needs parenting is rarely linear. It consists of ups and downs, twists and turns, and unexpected detours. Embracing these fluctuations with an open heart and a positive mindset is key to finding strength and perseverance amidst the challenges.

Strategies for Embracing the Journey:

1. **Practice Self-Compassion**: Be kind to yourself and recognize that it is natural to have difficult days. Give yourself grace and acknowledge that you are doing the best you can.

2. **Seek Support**: Connect with support groups or fellow parents on similar journeys. Sharing experiences and advice can help you feel less alone and more empowered.

3. **Focus on the Present**: Instead of worrying about the future or dwelling on the past, focus on the present moment. Celebrate small victories and cherish precious moments with your child.

4. **Stay Flexible**: Be open to adapting plans and strategies as needed. Flexibility allows you to navigate unexpected challenges with resilience.

5. **Practice Mindfulness**: Engage in mindfulness practices to stay centered and manage stress. Mindfulness can help you appreciate the beauty in every moment, no matter how challenging it may be.

6. **Celebrate Progress**: Recognize and celebrate the progress your child makes, no matter how small. Each step forward is a testament to their resilience and determination.

7. **Learn from Setbacks**: View setbacks as learning opportunities rather than failures. They can provide valuable insights into your child's needs and strengths.

8. **Remember Your Why**: Remind yourself of the love and commitment that led you to this journey.

Reconnect with your motivation during challenging times.

Embracing the journey's ups and downs allows you to cultivate a sense of gratitude and resilience, embracing each day with newfound strength and determination.

14.2 Celebrating Milestones and Achievements

In the journey of special needs parenting, celebrating milestones and achievements takes on profound significance. Every accomplishment, no matter how big or small, deserves recognition and celebration.

Ways to Celebrate Milestones:

1. **Personalize Celebrations**: Tailor celebrations to your child's interests and preferences. Whether it's a special outing, a favorite meal, or a small party with loved ones, make it meaningful to them.
2. **Document Progress**: Keep a journal or create a scrapbook to document your child's milestones and achievements. Looking back on these memories can fill your heart with joy and pride.
3. **Share Successes**: Share your child's successes with family and friends. Their encouragement and support will amplify the joy of the moment.

4. **Commemorate Efforts**: Celebrate the effort your child puts into their endeavors, regardless of the outcome. Effort and perseverance are worthy of celebration in themselves.

5. **Embrace Uniqueness**: Emphasize and celebrate your child's unique strengths and talents. Celebrations can be a beautiful expression of their individuality.

6. **Set Realistic Goals**: Set achievable goals for your child and celebrate when they reach them. Progress, no matter how gradual, is worth acknowledging.

7. **Create a "Wall of Achievements"**: Display your child's achievements in a designated space at home. This visual reminder of their growth and accomplishments can boost their self-esteem.

8. **Foster Peer Support**: Encourage peer support and recognition of each other's achievements among your child's friends or support groups.

Celebrating milestones and achievements instills a sense of accomplishment and self-worth in your child, motivating them to continue exploring their potential and reaching for their dreams.

14.3 Fostering Resilience in Both Parent and Child

Resilience is a valuable trait that allows both parent and child to navigate challenges and bounce back from adversity. Fostering resilience requires nurturing emotional well-being, fostering coping skills, and building a strong support system.

Strategies for Fostering Resilience:

1. **Practice Emotional Expression**: Encourage your child to express their emotions openly and without judgment. Create a safe space for them to share their feelings.

2. **Model Resilience**: Demonstrate resilience in your own life, showing your child that setbacks are a natural part of the journey and can be overcome.

3. **Encourage Problem-Solving**: Teach your child problem-solving skills, empowering them to face challenges with confidence.

4. **Build a Support Network**: Cultivate a strong support network of family, friends, and professionals who can offer guidance and encouragement.

5. **Encourage Healthy Coping Mechanisms**: Help your child discover healthy coping mechanisms, such as creative outlets, physical activities, or relaxation techniques.

6. **Foster a Growth Mindset**: Emphasize the importance of a growth mindset, where mistakes are opportunities to learn and grow.

7. **Cultivate Gratitude**: Encourage gratitude practices, helping your child focus on the positive aspects of their life.

8. **Seek Professional Help**: If needed, seek professional counseling or therapy for both parent and

child to develop coping strategies and emotional resilience.

By fostering resilience in both parent and child, you create a foundation of strength that allows your family to face challenges with courage and determination. Resilience enables you to embrace change, celebrate successes, and find joy in the journey of special needs parenting.

Overall, the journey of special needs parenting is a testament to love, strength, and unwavering dedication. Embracing change, celebrating successes, and fostering resilience are essential components of this extraordinary journey. Through ups and downs, challenges, and achievements, you have the opportunity to witness the incredible growth and potential of your child. Each milestone and success is a testament to their unique abilities and spirit.

As you continue on this journey, remember that you are not alone. Connect with others who share your journey and seek support when needed. Together, you can celebrate successes, navigate challenges, and create a nurturing environment that empowers your child to flourish and embrace their full potential.

May this journey be filled with joy, love, and boundless possibilities for you and your precious child. Embrace the moments of change, find inspiration in every milestone, and let resilience be the guiding light that illuminates your path toward a bright and promising future.

CONCLUSION

The journey of special needs parenting is a remarkable and transformative experience, filled with moments of joy, challenges, growth, and resilience. Throughout this book, we have explored various aspects of special needs parenting, delving into understanding special needs, early intervention, building a support network, creating an inclusive home environment, nurturing communication skills, finding the right educational setting, advocating for Individualized Education Plans (IEPs) and 504 Plans, supporting learning at home, prioritizing health and wellness, sensory integration and regulation, encouraging physical activity and recreation, and addressing legal and financial considerations.

We have also discussed the importance of embracing change, celebrating successes, and fostering resilience in both parent and child.

As you continue on this journey, remember that every child is unique, and there is no one-size-fits-all approach to special needs parenting. Embrace the diversity of experiences and find what works best for your family. Seek support, connect with other parents, and never hesitate to ask for help when needed.

Remember that being a special needs parent is a continuous learning process. Stay open to new ideas, strategies, and resources that can enrich your child's life and your own. Celebrate the milestones and achievements, no matter how small, and take pride in the progress your child makes.

To further support you on this journey, I have included several valuable resources in the appendices:

Appendix A: Resource Guide

In this appendix, you will find a compilation of resources, organizations, and websites that offer support, information, and services for families with special needs. From advocacy groups to therapeutic programs, this resource guide can be a valuable reference in your quest for information and assistance.

Please note that the resources listed here are not an exhaustive list, and the availability of services may vary depending on your location. You're encouraged to explore these resources and reach out to the organizations to find the most suitable support for your family's needs.

National Parent Organizations:
1. National Parent Center on Transition and Employment: A national center focused on assisting families in supporting their young adults with special needs in transitioning to adulthood and employment.
2. **Parent to Parent USA**: A national organization connecting parents of children with special needs to provide support and share experiences.

3. **Family Voices**: A national organization advocating for family-centered care, providing resources and support for families with children and youth with special healthcare needs.

Disability-Specific Organizations:

1. **Autism Speaks**: An organization dedicated to promoting autism awareness, funding research, and providing resources and support for individuals and families affected by autism spectrum disorders.
2. **Down Syndrome Association**: Various regional and national organizations that offer support, resources, and advocacy for individuals with Down syndrome and their families.
3. **Cerebral Palsy Foundation**: A nonprofit organization focusing on improving the lives of individuals with cerebral palsy through research, resources, and educational programs.
4. **National Association of the Deaf**: A civil rights organization that promotes the rights and accessibility of individuals who are deaf or hard of hearing.

Government Agencies:

1. **U.S. Department of Education**: Provides information and resources related to special education, the Individuals with Disabilities Education Act (IDEA), and parent involvement.
2. **Centers for Disease Control and Prevention (CDC)**: Offers resources and information on developmental milestones and disabilities.
3. **Social Security Administration**: Provides information about disability benefits, including Supplemental Security Income (SSI) and Social Security Disability Insurance (SSDI).

Education and Advocacy:

1. **Council for Exceptional Children (CEC):** A professional association for educators, providing resources and support for special education professionals and families.
2. **Wrightslaw**: A website offering information, resources, and legal guidance on special education law and advocacy.
3. **National Center for Learning Disabilities (NCLD):** An organization focused on supporting individuals with learning disabilities and their families through advocacy and resources.

Therapy and Medical Support:

- **American Physical Therapy Association (APTA)**: Offers resources and a directory to find physical therapists specializing in pediatric care.
- **American Occupational Therapy Association (AOTA)**: Provides resources and a directory to find occupational therapists specializing in pediatric care.
- **American Speech-Language-Hearing Association (ASHA)**: Offers resources and a directory to find speech-language pathologists specializing in pediatric care.

Technology and Accessibility:

1. The **National Center for Accessible Media (NCAM)**: Provides resources and information on accessible media and technology for individuals with disabilities.
2. **AbleData**: A database of assistive technology products and resources to enhance independence and accessibility.

Financial and Legal Assistance:

1. **Special Needs Alliance**: A network of attorneys specializing in special needs planning and advocacy.
2. **National Disability Institute**: Provides resources and information on financial planning for individuals with disabilities.
3. **Supplemental Nutrition Assistance Program (SNAP)**: A federal assistance program providing nutrition support to eligible low-income individuals and families.

Online Communities and Forums:

- **Parenting Special Needs Magazine**: An online magazine offering articles, resources, and a community for parents of children with special needs.
- **MySpecialNeedsNetwork**: An online platform providing resources and a supportive community for families of individuals with special needs.

Remember that each family's journey is unique, and the resources that best suit your needs may vary. Don't hesitate to reach out to local support groups, parent organizations, and educational institutions for additional resources and information. You are not alone on this journey, and the support and assistance available to you are vast.

I hope this resource guide serves as a valuable tool to empower and support you as you continue to navigate the beautiful and transformative path of special needs parenting.

Appendix B: Glossary of Terms

Navigating the world of special needs can sometimes involve encountering unfamiliar terms and jargon. This glossary of terms provides clear and concise explanations to help you better understand the language and terminology used in the context of special needs parenting.

1. **Individualized Education Plan (IEP)**: A legally binding document developed for students with disabilities that outlines the educational goals, services, accommodations, and support they will receive in the school setting.

2. **504 Plan**: A plan developed under Section 504 of the Rehabilitation Act of 1973, which provides accommodations and support to students with disabilities in general education settings to ensure equal access to education.

3. **Autism Spectrum Disorder (ASD)**: A developmental disorder characterized by challenges in social communication and interaction, restricted interests, and repetitive behaviors.

4. **Down Syndrome**: A genetic disorder caused by the presence of an extra copy of chromosome 21, leading to developmental delays, intellectual disabilities, and characteristic physical features.

5. **Cerebral Palsy**: A group of neurological disorders affecting movement, muscle tone, and

posture, often caused by brain damage occurring before, during, or shortly after birth.

6. **Developmental Delay**: A significant lag in reaching developmental milestones compared to typical developmental timelines.

7. **Speech-Language Pathologist (SLP)**: A professional who assesses and treats speech and language disorders in children and adults.

8. **Occupational Therapist (OT)**: A professional who helps individuals develop the skills necessary for daily living and self-care activities.

9. **Physical Therapist (PT)**: A professional who assesses and treats movement and physical impairments.

10. **Sensory Processing Disorder (SPD)**: A condition where the brain has difficulty receiving and responding to sensory information, leading to challenges in processing sensory stimuli.

11. **Inclusion**: The practice of integrating individuals with disabilities into mainstream settings, such as classrooms and community activities, to promote equal opportunities and social interaction.

12. **Assistive Technology**: Devices, tools, or software designed to support individuals with disabilities in performing tasks and activities.

13. **Transition Planning**: The process of preparing individuals with disabilities for adulthood, including post-secondary education, employment, and independent living.

14. **Behavioral Intervention**: Strategies and approaches used to address challenging

behaviors and promote positive behaviors in individuals with special needs.

15. **Individual Family Service Plan (IFSP)**: A written plan developed for infants and toddlers with developmental delays and disabilities, outlining early intervention services and family support.

16. **Special Education**: Educational programs and services designed to meet the unique needs of students with disabilities.

17. **Inclusive Classroom**: A classroom setting where students with and without disabilities learn together with appropriate support and accommodations.

18. **Augmentative and Alternative Communication (AAC)**: Systems and methods used to support or replace speech for individuals with communication challenges.

19. **Respite Care**: Temporary care and support provided to individuals with disabilities to give their primary caregivers a break.

20. **Developmental Pediatrician**: A medical doctor specializing in the assessment and management of developmental and behavioral issues in children.

Remember that this glossary provides only brief definitions for key terms. The world of special needs is vast and diverse, and definitions may vary depending on the context and individual circumstances. If you encounter unfamiliar terms or have questions about specific concepts, don't hesitate to reach out to professionals, educators, or support organizations for clarification and guidance.

Appendix C: Recommended Reading

Knowledge is a powerful tool for understanding and supporting your child's needs. In this appendix, is a compiled list of recommended reading materials, including books, articles, and publications, that cover a wide range of topics related to special needs parenting, advocacy, education, and more.

1. "**The Spark**: A Mother's Story of Nurturing, Genius, and Autism" by Kristine Barnett
2. "**Uniquely Human**: A Different Way of Seeing Autism" by Barry M. Prizant, Ph.D.
3. "**Far From the Tree**: Parents, Children, and the Search for Identity" by Andrew Solomon
4. "**The Out-of-Sync Child**: Recognizing and Coping with Sensory Processing Disorder" by Carol Kranowitz
5. "**No Drama Discipline**: The Whole-Brain Way to Calm the Chaos and Nurture Your Child's Developing Mind" by Daniel J. Siegel and Tina Payne Bryson
6. "**The Explosive Child**: A New Approach for Understanding and Parenting Easily Frustrated, Chronically Inflexible Children" by Ross W. Greene, Ph.D.
7. "**The Special Needs Parent Handbook**: Critical Strategies and Practical Advice to Help You Survive and Thrive" by Jonathan L. Singer, Ph.D., and Karen L. Sewell, Ph.D.

8. **"Wrightslaw**: From Emotions to Advocacy: The Special Education Survival Guide" by Pam Wright and Pete Wright

9. **"Raising a Sensory Smart Child**: The Definitive Handbook for Helping Your Child with Sensory Processing Issues" by Lindsey Biel and Nancy Peske

10. **"Neurotribes**: The Legacy of Autism and the Future of Neurodiversity" by Steve Silberman

These recommended reading materials provide a diverse and enriching array of perspectives on special needs parenting and related topics. Each book offers valuable insights, strategies, and emotional support for parents and caregivers.

Note: Book availability may vary based on location and publication date. Some titles may also be available in digital formats or audiobooks for added accessibility.

I hope that this book has provided you with valuable insights, practical tips, and a sense of encouragement in your special needs parenting journey. You are not alone in this experience, and with love, dedication, and support, your child will thrive and embrace their unique potential.

Thank you for embarking on this journey with me. May your family be filled with love, joy, and boundless possibilities as you continue to navigate the beautiful and transformative path of special needs parenting.

ACKNOWLEDGMENTS

Writing this book, "Beyond Boundaries: 101 Practical Tips for Special Needs Parenting," has been a labor of love and a collective effort. I would like to take this opportunity to express my heartfelt gratitude to all those who have contributed to the creation of this valuable resource.

First and foremost, I want to thank all the parents and caregivers of children with special needs. Your dedication, strength, and unwavering love for your children have been a true inspiration. Your experiences and stories have shaped the content of this book, and I hope it serves as a source of support and guidance in your parenting journey.

I am deeply thankful to the professionals, educators, and therapists who have devoted their expertise and time to enriching the lives of children with special needs. Your valuable insights and knowledge have been invaluable in shaping the advice and tips shared in this book.

I extend my gratitude to all the individuals and organizations that provided valuable resources and information for the resource guide in Appendix A. Your commitment to supporting families with special needs is commendable, and I am grateful for your contributions.

I would like to acknowledge the team of editors and reviewers who diligently worked to ensure the accuracy and clarity of the content. Your thoughtful feedback and expertise have been instrumental in shaping this book into its final form.

Finally, I would like to thank my family, friends, and loved ones for their unwavering support and encouragement throughout this endeavor. Your belief in me has been a driving force in bringing this book to fruition.

To all those who have contributed to the making of this book, directly or indirectly, I extend my heartfelt gratitude. It is my sincere hope that "Beyond Boundaries: 101 Practical Tips for Special Needs Parenting" becomes a valuable resource for families, providing guidance, support, and inspiration on the beautiful and rewarding journey of special needs parenting.

With gratitude,

Brenda Maye

www.ingramcontent.com/pod-product-compliance
Lightning Source LLC
Chambersburg PA
CBHW070852260726
48661CB00004B/1370